An Introduction to
Child Psychiatry

An Introduction to
Child Psychiatry
second edition

By STELLA CHESS, M.D.

Associate Professor of Psychiatry, New York University Medical Center; Associate Visiting Psychiatrist, Bellevue Hospital. Formerly Director of Child Psychiatry, New York Medical College; Psychiatrist-in-Charge, Child Guidance Clinic, and Chief Psychiatrist, Mental Retardation Clinic, Flower-Fifth Avenue Hospital; Visiting Psychiatrist, Bird S. Coler and Metropolitan Hospitals.

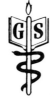

GRUNE & STRATTON

New York   and   London

Printed in U.S.A.
(PC-B)

Contents

Preface

THIS SECOND EDITION of *An Introduction to Child Psychiatry* is more than an updating of the first, which appeared ten years ago. It also reflects a somewhat different approach to the material, and each chapter accordingly has undergone substantial rewriting. Instead of offering a comprehensive survey of the subject—other texts have done this in the past few years—I have written a more personal document emphasizing concepts and techniques that I have found productive in my own clinical and research experience. I have dealt in detail with issues that often receive only brief mention but which I consider essential for a sound orientation to diagnosis and therapy.

The reader will note, for example, that the discussion focuses on the role of temperament in the interaction between the child and his environment. The recurrence of this theme does not mean I regard temperament as more important than such issues as motivation or parental influences. Rather, this emphasis seems useful because it is only in recent years that the significance of temperament in psychologic development has come to be appreciated. The contribution of temperament to normal and abnormal behavior has not been explained in detail in other child psychiatry texts.

The reader will also note that the concepts of community psychiatry recur in this book, even though there is no special section devoted to this subject. I believe it is unwise to deal with community psychiatry as if it were a separate technique. Community psychiatry involves all the relationships with schools, pediatric clinics, recreation centers, baby health stations, and community agencies that are relevant in case finding, diagnostic understanding, and treatment efforts calling for environmental manipulation.

Much that is presented in the following pages about diagnosis and treatment is directed toward students of psychiatry who are making their first excursions into the realm of human behavior from infancy through adolescence. However, I have tried to discuss each topic in a manner that would be understandable and meaningful to all who are professionally involved in the care of children with disturbances in mental or emotional functioning. For this reason, I have attempted wherever possible to avoid technical psychiatric terminology and complex theoretical formulations. My own teaching experience in child psychiatry has convinced me of both the possibility and desirability of using such simplified formulations in the training of psychiatrists as well as other professional personnel.

If this book provides its readers with a practical approach to child psychiatry, and with a key to the understanding of its more specialized literature, it will have accomplished its objective.

In acknowledging my debt to those who have helped me, I will not attempt to name everyone who made valuable comments or assisted in the technical preparation of the book. I would be remiss, however, if I failed to express appreciation for the contribution made by my editor, Dr. Samuel Sillen, whose insistence on clarity was uncompromising. I am also grateful to Mrs. Abby Hand for her editorial assistance. Not to be underestimated is the influence of my husband, Dr. Alexander Thomas, whose lack of shyness in making critical comments on the manuscript led to the tightening of many formulations.

STELLA CHESS, M.D.
New York City

1. The Role of Child Psychiatry

CHILD PSYCHIATRY plays a dual role today in the field of clinical medicine. While it has made rapid headway during the past generation as a discrete subspecialty, it has also been permeating general psychiatry, neurology and pediatrics as an indispensable part of these disciplines. Any survey of child psychiatry in the United States, however brief, must examine it within both these perspectives.

Development of the Subspecialty

The history of child psychiatry, like that of general psychiatry, has been influenced by developments outside the sphere of medicine. The introductory chapters in this history were written shortly after the turn of the century, when the psychoanalytic concept of childhood as the point of origin of many of the emotional problems besetting adults began to be reflected in psychiatric literature. Adolf Meyer's (1915) psychobiologic approach to the growth of personality and his appeals to psychiatrists to concern themselves with the study and treatment of emotionally ill children were also attracting professional attention. Concurrently, voluntary mental hygiene associations were stimulating public interest in the newer and more hopeful theories about the treatability of psychiatric disorders, and a series of sociopsychologic programs for their prevention or early treatment was being initiated by the child guidance movement.

During that period, the child guidance clinic was virtually the only setting in which the child psychiatrist functioned. In fact, the early history of child psychiatry in the United States is essentially that of the establishment and development of such clinics. Many years were to elapse before child psychiatry acquired appropriate recognition and professional status as a subspecialty of general psychiatry.

The first child guidance clinic was established in Chicago in 1909 for the express purpose of investigating the antecedents of juvenile delinquency. William Healy (1915), its organizer, went about this task by conducting diagnostic studies of individual delinquents referred by the Chicago Juvenile Court to his center, the Juvenile Psychopathic Institute. Prior to its establishment, aside from a relatively small number of children suffering from psychoses who were institutionalized in public or private mental hospitals, the only mentally deviant youngsters under psychiatric study were the feebleminded. Lightner Witmer's psychologic clinic, founded in 1896 at the University of Pennsylvania, was primarily concerned with the study, treatment and training of the feebleminded, and H. H. Goddard (1914) was also working with feebleminded children in a research laboratory opened in 1906 at the Vineland Training School in New Jersey. Although Witmer's clinic was actually the birthplace of child guidance and of organized clinical psychology in the United States, it played a less influential role in both fields and in the development of child psychiatry than the Juvenile Psychopathic Institute and similar clinics set up later in other cities, particularly the Judge Baker Foundation in Boston.

At a time when general psychiatry was largely concerned with institutional treatment and nosology, Healy's approach to delinquency was psychodynamic. His case methods provided for medical examinations and psychologic tests, but he focused on the noxious aspects of the delinquent's socioeconomic environment and on his emotional conflicts and personality difficulties. Healy, who later became a psychoanalyst, spoke of "mental analysis" in connection with his early researches. The youngsters he interviewed were invited to tell their "own story," an innovation which attracted much attention. Multiple causative factors in delinquency emerged from his analytic study of some 800 cases, reviewed in his mammoth textbook, *The Individual Delinquent*. This was one of many publications by Healy which stressed the need for individual psychotherapy to uncover and resolve the delinquent's psychopathology.

A new era of psychiatric case study was initiated with the exhaustive reports on delinquents gathered by Healy and his associates. The psychiatric hospitals, few of which had been taking detailed histories of individual patients, began to adopt the same practice more generally and also to explore the adverse social and environmental factors implicated in the breakdowns of their patients. Psychologists and social workers were included on the staffs of both the Boston Psychopathic Hospital, opened in 1912, and the Phipps Psychiatric Clinic, established a year later in Baltimore under the direction of Adolf Meyer. The outpatient departments of both institutions, and, beginning in 1915, that of the Allentown State Hospital in Pennsylvania, admitted youngsters with various types of psychiatric disorders.

Studies of the psychologic development of children, first organized at the Yale Clinic of Child Development in 1911 by Arnold Gesell, were also undertaken by other child study centers. The emphasis in these exploratory studies, as in those made in Healy's clinic, was on diagnostic evaluation of the children's disorders.

The epidemic of *encephalitis lethargica* following World War I created a pressing need for psychiatric facilities for the large number of youngsters with behavior disorders consequent to the disease. Inpatient services were created to care for them. These included the children's departments at Bellevue Hospital and Kings Park State Hospital in New York as well as the Franklin School in Philadelphia during its eleven years of existence.

Another milestone in residential treatment was August Aichhorn's work with delinquent adolescents in Vienna following World War I. This initial attempt to apply psychoanalytic principles to the inpatient treatment of children aroused much interest in the United States after Aichhorn's book on the experiment, with an introduction by Sigmund Freud, was published in Austria in 1925. An English translation was subsequently issued in this country under the title *Wayward Youth* (1935).

Of extreme importance for the development of child psychiatry in this country was the nationwide mushrooming of child guidance clinics which began in 1922. This resulted from a comprehensive long range program directed by the National Committee for Mental Hygiene and subsidized by the Commonwealth Fund for more than a decade. Although launched specifically for the "prevention of delinquency," this undertaking turned out to have a much broader significance. Demonstration child guidance clinics were conducted for a five-year period in many cities throughout the country. The demonstration program was followed by the establish-

ment of a center for the training of psychiatrists, psychologists and
students entering the field of psychiatric social work. This center,
located in New York and known as the Institute for Child Guidance,
remained in existence for six years. Like the demonstration clinics, it
concentrated on training professional personnel for the child guidance clinics and on developing and systematizing treatment techniques. Over a period of years, too, many psychiatrists were trained
in this new field under fellowships provided largely by the Commonwealth Fund and the Rockefeller Foundation.

The founding of the American Orthopsychiatric Association in
1924 served to unite organizationally the members of the three
disciplines which were then beginning to function as the clinic
treatment team—psychiatrists, psychologists and psychiatric social
workers. The overwhelming majority of the psychiatrists instru-
mental in setting up the Association worked in the fields of child
guidance, delinquency and mental hygiene. Hence, therapeutic
prevention, training programs, and the development of treatment
techniques for the community clinics received major attention in
the meetings of the AOA. Under its auspices, the directors of child
guidance clinics met regularly, using these meetings as a sort of
clearing house for their activities. These "director's meetings"
ultimately led to the formation of a separate organization, the
American Association of Psychiatric Clinics for Children. This
voluntary association, organized in 1946, has played an influential
role in setting standards for its member clinics.

The original function of the child guidance clinic, as has been
pointed out, was to conduct diagnostic studies and make recommendations for treatment. Treatment in the first clinics encom-
passed little more than suggestions for the resolution or alleviation
of a child's environmental or social difficulties. Transformation of
the child guidance clinic into a facility oriented to more direct and
intensive treatment, especially psychotherapy, was basically accomplished during the decade of the thirties.

Many factors contributed to this transformation. Various follow-
up studies had already brought to light serious shortcomings in the
diagnostic study as well as in the treatment program recommended
to the outside agency or parent referring a case. All too often, the
source of the referral failed to carry out the recommendations made
because it was either unable or unwilling to do so. Furthermore,

leaders in the child guidance movement had long sensed the need for a shift in emphasis from diagnosis to psychotherapy, the latter to embody the latest concepts in child psychiatry and to be provided by the clinic itself.

The change-over was facilitated by the availability of a substantial number of European-trained and analytically oriented psychotherapists for treatment, training and supervisory posts in guidance clinics. Some were distinguished European psychoanalysts who had come to this country as anti-Nazi refugees. American medical students who had gone abroad for special training in psychotherapy and child analysis, many as Commonwealth Fund Fellows, also contributed significantly to the development and expansion of the treatment programs.

From this time on, diagnostic study tended to be relegated to a subordinate position, although the approach to it has continued to vary considerably from clinic to clinic, depending on the particular orientation of the psychiatric supervisors. Some clinics regard diagnosis as of little or no importance. Others see the diagnostic process as simply a preliminary to treatment, a passageway which must be crossed by the child en route to the treatment setting. Still other clinics adhere to the concept that what is formulated during the processing of a new case is little more than a working hypothesis and that the diagnosis itself is actually made during the early stages of treatment.

Outside as well as inside the child guidance clinic, the decade of the thirties initiated significant developments in child psychiatry. Children's units were established in several psychiatric hospitals, the first two being opened at the Allentown State Hospital and at the Rockland State Hospital in Orangeburg, New York. New residential centers for emotionally disturbed youngsters requiring inpatient treatment were founded by charitable groups and other agencies, including university medical centers.

The subsequent development of residential treatment services has reflected the growing recognition that disturbed children require a milieu and treatment program oriented to their own special needs. The emergence in inpatient residential facilities of such a "total treatment approach"—the use of the "controlled living" setting around the clock to supplement the regular therapy program—has tended to increase the natural divergence in treatment philosophies and procedures between the psychiatrists functioning in these services and those providing ambulatory treatment in guidance clinics or in the relatively new field of private practice.

A program of close collaboration between psychiatrists and pediatricians inaugurated at the Johns Hopkins University Hospital in 1930 was probably the first formal recognition accorded child psychiatry by a medical teaching center in this country. Children's psychiatric units were gradually introduced in this and many other university medical centers in much the same way as child psychiatry was introduced into their curricula: that is, as a responsibility of the department of medicine, neurology or general psychiatry.

Since the passage of the National Mental Health Act in 1946, federal funds have been made available yearly for advanced training and research in child psychiatry. The National Institute of Mental Health, which administers the stipends, fellowships, and other types of grants made to individuals and institutions, also carries on research in children's psychiatric disorders at its own Laboratory of Child Research in Bethesda, Maryland.

The pioneering efforts of the directors of child guidance clinics and of various professional bodies to determine the basic qualifications, training requirements, and other conditions that should govern such practice culminated in the creation of the American Academy of Child Psychiatry. The Academy was founded in 1952 for the purpose of promoting the study and treatment of the psychiatric problems of children, and launched its own journal, *The Journal of the Academy of Child Psychiatry,* as an important outlet for theoretic, clinical and research studies.

Child Psychiatry in the Other Specialties

As a member of a closely related group of specialists, the child psychiatrist has to keep in touch with significant developments in general psychiatry, neurology and pediatrics. In turn, the general psychiatrist, neurologist and pediatrician are confronted in their professional spheres with problems requiring a fundamental knowledge of the nature and treatment of psychiatric disorders arising in the early years of life.

In General Psychiatry

In treating adults, the psychiatrist often deals with the effects of interpersonal relationships and traumatizing events in the childhood of his patients. During therapy, inferences are drawn about parental attitudes experienced by the patient as a child, especially with respect to neurotic defense mechanisms that may have been initiated or strengthened by these attitudes. The psychiatrist frequently finds it necessary to distinguish between situations in which the patient was fortuitously exposed to such destructive attitudes and those in which he was already manifesting behavioral disturbances that were contributing to destructive interaction. For this reason alone, it is essential that the general psychiatrist clearly understand the nature of childhood disturbances and, especially, the memory distortions to which they may give rise. An adult's recollection of childhood may mislead the clinician unless he is aware that an event might not have occurred as the patient recalls it.

If the adult patient is a parent, the possibility that his behavior may undermine the emotional development of his offspring becomes a matter of concern to his psychiatrist. To deal with this possibility appropriately requires an appreciation of the effects of parent-child interaction on a child's functioning.

Often, an adult patient is worried about some aspect of his youngster's behavior and wishes to know if it has any pathologic significance and if additional aid seems to be indicated. Rather than advising a complete diagnostic work-up by a child psychiatrist each time he has to handle such inquiries, the general psychiatrist does better to maintain his footing in the area of child behavior in order to deal with such questions in a discriminating and appropriate manner. For example, when the adult patient is airing his own resentments about the parental treatment he recalls having received in his childhood, the psychiatrist can use the occasion to help clarify such issues as sibling rivalry, appropriate discipline, or the proper balance between authoritativeness and permissiveness. Advice on such matters, however, must be grounded in knowledge if the practitioner is to merit the confidence placed in him by the patient.

Some familiarity with the procedures of the child psychiatrist often proves helpful to the general psychiatrist who is unaccustomed to young patients but is called upon to deal with them from time to time. Otherwise, for example, after suggesting that the youngster being studied draw a picture, the clinician may be embarrassed to discover that he is short of ideas on how to get a meaningful discussion under way. He may also have a tendency to brush aside as trivia an adolescent girl's chatter about boys or a schoolboy's complaints that his teacher blames him for all the noise in his classroom or that his playmates are picking on him for no reason whatsoever. Even if the practitioner is fully aware of the significance of such statements, he may want to know how to use play as a mode of communication, or how to determine whether a pattern of behavior is characteristic of a child or reflects special tensions created by the interview situation.

In Neurology

The neurologist called upon to diagnose children often finds that competence in system-by-system testing does not, in itself, insure adequate examination of a youngster who is frightened or hyperactive, or who, for some reason, is unable to follow directions. Skill and imagination may be required on the part of the neurologist to transform his procedures into games or, perhaps, to disguise them, and to maintain a sufficiently friendly and casual manner to put the child at ease. Some knowledge of child behavior and of behavioral problems is helpful in these situations.

The neurologic examination of young children presents special problems. As Paine and Oppé (1966) point out, it is more difficult to decide whether or not a given finding is abnormal in children than it is in adults. "The range of variation of normal is greater among children," these authors observe, "and the number of standards which must be learnt in order to evaluate the function of the nervous system at all the ages from the newborn period to adolescence is far greater than the changes which occur from adolescence to old age. Many special responses and automatisms are peculiar to early childhood and these responses are constantly changing with increasing age, as some disappear and others become demonstrable for the first time."

An understanding of these developmental sequences is essential for assessing the significance of deviations from the norm. Although neurologic examinations of infants are not yet highly predictive, they provide the diagnostician with valuable and often indispensable information.

Increasing awareness of the specific neurologic problems found in children gave rise to the new subspecialty of pediatric neurology, which has made much progress in recent years. This field is now officially recognized as a subspecialty with its own certifying examination given by the American Board of Psychiatry and Neurology.

In Pediatrics

Far more often than the general psychiatrist and the neurologist, the pediatrician is called upon to step across the boundary of his specialty into the territory of the child behaviorist. The American parent, especially one in the income bracket that can afford the services of a private pediatrician, is less content than in the past with mere decrees on when an infant should be weaned or toilet-trained, for instance. Increasingly attentive to her child's emotional development, the mother today wants the pediatrician to explain and discuss his recommendations. He is expected to know what psychologic effects different schedules and modes of training will have on her child's maturation, and perhaps even to answer any questions in her mind about interpersonal relationships and the latest theories about hostility, motility, and the like.

The child psychiatrist would like to attribute this metamorphosis in pediatric practice to his own constructive influence, but over the years other developments have also contributed to the changing character of pediatric service. A major factor was the introduction of antibiotics, which sharply reduced the incidence of pneumonia, mastoiditis, rheumatic carditis and similar childhood diseases. Time and energy formerly needed to deal with physical pathology can now be devoted to problems of personality development. Hence, a pediatrician may be seeking the kind of knowledge that will enable him to deal almost as competently with night fears and dependency reactions as with measles, middle-ear infections and allergies. He will wish to understand the psychodynamics of certain feeding problems and to know how to distinguish between behavior traits that are likely to be outgrown and those that may form the nucleus for serious disturbance in later life if not properly dealt with at once. He needs to know how to reassure when reassurance is in order and also how to mobilize a parent into immediate action when this is what the situation requires.

The psychologically oriented pediatrician is in a position to function as a preventive psychiatrist. Since he observes behavior patterns in their formative stages, it is possible for him to either encourage or discourage the development of particular trends. It is he who usually has the first opportunity to recognize the emergence of destructive patterns of behavior, such as morbid dependence, self-depreciation or unhealthy expressions of hostility. Within the context of his regular professional contacts with parents, the pediatrician is often able to make them aware that their attitudes are overanxious or overpermissive. Whether or not a particular effort at preventive therapy on the part of the pediatrician proves to be fruitful, it must be based on sound knowledge of the dynamics of the parent-child relationship and the relative strength of the negative and positive forces with which he has to work.

The Child Psychiatrist's Relationships With Other Specialties

The child psychiatrist, for equally cogent reasons, has to keep au courant of developments in general psychiatry, neurology and pediatrics.

With General Psychiatry

Although the subject of the child psychiatrist's diagnostic evaluation and treatment is a child, the complaint and initial evidence of the patient's presumed disorder are presented by adults, usually one or both parents. In addition to taking part in the discussion of causative factors and other circumstances surrounding a child's illness, the parents must be entrusted with carrying out whatever recommendations are made. Thus, sensitivity and therapeutic skill in dealing with adults are obviously required of the child psychiatrist even though he does not enter into a true treatment relationship with adults.

The child psychiatrist must try to determine how objective the adults are in their reporting of problems and whether they are capable of forming good relationships with the child. The clinician dealing with a child is also concerned with the quality of the parents' relationship to each other and, especially, with their ability to carry out both the letter and the spirit of instructions. He must, in other words, be able to recognize deviant personality and marked neurotic trends as well as a vast assortment of relatively normal characterologic traits in the adults closest to his youthful patient.

In the continuing process of working with parents, the best results are achieved when the child psychiatrist underscores the positive elements of their personalities, takes due account of their anxieties, and remains fully aware of the areas in which their interaction with the child is apt to be destructive. The child psychiatrist must be aware that recognition of morbid psychiatric tendencies in a parent is a signal to desist from making a suggestion which might tend to threaten an already tenuous adjustment.

With Pediatrics

The child psychiatrist also needs to keep his knowledge of pediatrics up to date. It is now recognized that organic difficulties may play a far greater role in the genesis of psychiatric disorders than was previously suspected, and the relationship between physical illness and disturbance in behavior is becoming more obvious. To understand fully the effect which a particular physical illness may have on behavior requires, first of all, a familiarity with pediatric disease syndromes. The child's capacity to make a good adjustment to the stress or after-effects of a physical condition, or the ability of a parent to handle it constructively, cannot be determined until the nature of the medical condition itself is fully understood.

The child psychiatrist must be equally aware of the effect that a past illness and its treatment may have on the child's behavior. Very often, the treatment necessary for certain illnesses may set up a strain between parent and child. Allergy treatment, for example, which often involves severe restrictions on a child's diet or exposure to pets, may set up a chain reaction of parent-child conflict and hostility, whose end result may persist long after the allergy, and with it the need for restriction, has disappeared. If this is realized by the psychiatrist, he will avoid a mistaken judgment as to the cause of parent-child conflict.

An understanding of pediatrics may alert the psychiatrist to signs of physical illness in a child who has been brought to him for treatment of behavior problems. Such an illness may previously have been unsuspected by the child's parents or wrongly interpreted by them as a purely emotional disturbance. This was strikingly illustrated, in my own experience, by the case of an eight year old boy brought in by his parents for treatment of a behavior problem and characterized by them as "kid passive resistance." His passivity and constant avoidance of activities requiring coordination turned out to be a sign of amyotonia with superimposed secondary emotional disorder.

In psychiatric practice, the question often arises whether some physical disease is directly responsible for behavioral symptoms or whether the latter represent a secondary behavior disorder arising in reaction to the illness or the treatment procedures applied. In many baffling situations, it is impossible to formulate an adequate treatment plan until such a distinction has been made. The child psychiatrist who has to rely wholly on the opinions and reports of others about a pediatric condition may discover that there are legitimate differences of opinion between experts on issues crucial to the diagnosis of the behavior. Consequently, it is desirable that the psychiatrist possess the knowledge necessary to evaluate for himself, to some extent, at least, fundamental facts in a pediatric picture.

The need for better communication between the two specialties has recently been emphasized by leading pediatricians and child psychiatrists (Eisenberg, 1967; Lourie, 1966; Richmond, 1967; Senn, 1946). Too often, the pediatrician does not receive reports from the psychiatrist to whom he has referred a case. When he does get reports, they are apt to be couched in psychiatric jargon that he may too easily dismiss as beyond his ken or as irrelevant. On the other hand, the psychiatrist depends on the pediatrician's full cooperation in providing a clear picture of the child's physical history.

Emerging concepts of community mental health care suggest the need to revise the traditional approaches embodied in most child guidance centers. Too often the medical history of a child is not taken in such centers, since it is assumed that children with important medical defects are cared for elsewhere. If such children do arrive at a child guidance clinic they are likely to be screened out and referred to another center. In contrast, one may cite the psychiatric unit of the Bellevue Hospital Pediatric Outpatient Department (Chess and Lyman, 1969). Here the child is seen by both a pediatrician who identifies a behavior disorder and a psychiatrist who has a direct opportunity to discuss the child's physical state and to obtain further data. The two specialists become active colleagues, pooling their skills to help the patient.

With Neurology

Assessment of a child's neurologic state is often an indispensable aspect of a diagnostic study. In the course of taking a history, the psychiatrist may become alerted to the possibility that there is impairment of the child's central nervous system even though the history provides no evidence of fetal damage or childhood illness. A child's difficulties in coordination or perception, or his passive or anxious approach to some motor activity, for example, may indicate brain damage which was either too obscure or diffuse to have gained diagnostic recognition earlier.

The child psychiatrist who maintains his knowledge of neurology can, by asking detailed questions, pursue his own inquiry into possible difficulties of this nature and also do a brief neurologic examination himself. How intense a neurologic investigation is required for a particular child is something the psychiatrist must be able to determine on the basis of his own training in neurology. When a more thorough examination by a pediatric neurologist is needed, his services will be put to better use if the child psychiatrist can discuss with him the implications of conclusive findings and evaluate any that are inconclusive. Interpretations of such laboratory tests as electroencephalograms, in particular, are not always clearcut. To weigh such findings adequately, in terms of the total clinical picture, one must keep abreast of developments in the field of neurology.

The child psychiatrist, then, must approach any problem presented to him not as a member of an isolated specialty but as a medical practitioner deeply aware of the relevance of many other aspects of clinical knowledge to his own particular area.

SELECTED REFERENCES

Aichhorn, A.: *Wayward Youth*. New York, Viking, 1935.

Chess, S., and Lyman, M.: A psychiatric unit in a general hospital pediatric clinic. *Amer. J. Orthopsychiat.* 39:77-85, 1969.

Eisenberg, L.: The relationship between psychiatry and pediatrics: A disputatious view. *Pediatrics* 39:645-647, 1967.

Glueck, S., and Glueck, E. T.: *One Thousand Juvenile Delinquents.* Cambridge, Harvard University Press, 1934.

Goddard, H. H.: *School Training of Defective Children.* Yonkers, World Book Co., 1914.

Healy, W.: *The Individual Delinquent.* Boston, Little, Brown, 1915.

Kanner, L.: *A History of the Care and Study of the Mentally Retarded.* Springfield, Ill., Charles C Thomas, 1964.

Lourie, R. S.: Problems of diagnosis and treatment: Communication between pediatrician and psychiatrist. *Pediatrics* 37:1000, 1966.

Lowrey, L. G., and Sloane, V.: *Orthopsychiatry, 1923-1948—Retrospect and Prospect.* New York, American Orthopsychiatric Association, 1948.

Meyer, A.: The justification of psychobiology as a topic of the medical curriculum. *Psychol. Bull.* 12:328, 1915.

Paine, R. S., and Oppé, T. E.: *Neurological Examination of Children.* London, William Heinemann, 1966.

Richmond, J. B.: Child development: A basic science for pediatrics. *Pediatrics* 39:649-658, 1967.

Senn, M. J. E.: Relationship of pediatrics and psychiatry. *Amer. J. Dis. Child.* 71:537-549, 1946.

2. The Child as a Developing Organism

THE GROWING CHILD has been studied within many different theoretic frameworks. Various schools of thought have found the key to development in tactics of adaptation, motives and drive states, environmental influences, and organic determinants. Some theorists focus on the orderly progress of physiologic maturation, others on the satisfaction or frustration of instinctual needs, and still others on overt behavior to the exclusion of intrapsychic processes. No single approach, however, fully explains the richness and diversity of human personality.

The Concept of Interaction

Historically, the theorists have been divided into two major camps: the "constitutionalists" and the "environmentalists." The constitutionalist view attributes psychologic differences to inborn physical or physiologic characteristics. This position may be traced as far back as Hippocrates, who classified four types of personality based on differences in their "body humors." In the twentieth century, the constitutional approach is exemplified in the work of Kretschmer (1925) in Germany and Sheldon (1940) in the United States. These investigators identify various body types and link them to specific personality characteristics.

While the constitutionalist view calls attention to the important role of physiologic factors, it oversimplifies the issue by assuming that physical makeup as such is the main causative element in the unfolding of personality. Complex personality structures and elaborate psychopathologic syndromes are reduced to genetically determined patterns of organization.

The constitutionalist approach dominated psychiatric thought in the nineteenth century, and was reflected in the popular concept that mental illnesses were inherited through a "bad seed." Many types of abnormal behavior were attributed to "constitutional weak-

15

ness." In general, environment was considered to have little influence on a person's "inner" development.

This static and fatalistic view of "human nature" clashed with an increasing body of scientific evidence that many traits once considered hereditary are largely the result of experience. The work of Freud (1924), Pavlov (1927), and Watson (1925) in the early decades of this century focused attention on the environmental determinants of development. While representing different viewpoints, all three men were influential in discrediting the constitutionalist position.

Psychoanalytic theory, despite its basic assumption of biologic drives and instincts, assigns primary importance to the early environmental influences that are thought to direct and fix the specific forms and object relationships of the libido. Freud's clinical studies convinced him that the adult personality reflects the motives and attitudes of the parents and the kind of care given in early life. Most psychoanalytic studies of early child development have concentrated on the determining role of the parents, especially the mother. Thus, such workers as Levy (1943), Ribble (1943), Anna Freud (1948), and Bowlby (1951) have assigned prime importance in the child's development to intrafamilial phenomena as manifested during the first years of life.

Another group of psychoanalytically oriented investigators, going beyond the intrafamilial components, have emphasized the importance of social and cultural influences in shaping the child's development. This group includes such influential contemporary writers as Kardiner (1945), Erikson (1950), and Fromm (1955).

The work of Pavlov contributed to environmentalism from a different direction. Pavlov's approach was primarily experimental and physiologic. He profoundly influenced concepts of development by demonstrating that conditioned reflexes are the basis for complex habits and behavior patterns.

The role of learning mechanisms in development was also emphasized by Watson (1925), founder of the school of behaviorism. Believing that planned habit training could mold the child in any desired direction, he wrote: "Give me a dozen healthy infants, well-formed, and my own specified world to bring them up in, and I'll guarantee to take any one at random and train him to become any type of specialist I might select—doctor, lawyer, artist, merchant-chief, and yes, even beggarman and thief, regardless of his talents, penchants, tendencies, abilities, vocations, and race of his ancestors." Watson's oversimplified view left out of account the influence of differences in the individual capacities of children and their reactions to environment. As our knowledge of the learning process has grown it has become increasingly difficult to apply any simple concept to the development of the child.

Another line of investigation was developed by Gesell (1943), who described stages of behavior and development in children. He based his behavior calendar on observation of groups of children at various age levels, beginning with infancy. Gesell concluded that physiologic and behavioral growth proceeds at a certain pace and that behavior at any age is an expression of the child's state of maturity and adaptation to the environment.

A similar emphasis on general developmental features is found in the influential studies by Piaget (1959) on the growth of reason in children. When can they grasp cause and effect? When can they make abstract judgments? When and how do they achieve mastery of mathematical processes? Piaget observes that these intellectual functions seem to develop by orderly stages and sequences.

Thus, our concepts of the forces operating in the child's development have been enlarged from many directions. Freud called attention to the emotional and motivational factors involved in early parent-child relationships. The culturalists emphasized the important influence of society at large. Pavlov demonstrated the conditioned reflex and its place in patterning behavior. Watson and the later learning theorists explored the role that training and learning play in determining behavior patterns. Gesell's work called attention to the schedule of neurologic and behavioral maturation, while Piaget showed that cognitive functions have their own sequential course of growth.

Increasingly, serious workers in psychiatry and psychology have come to recognize that both normal development and disturbances in development, instead of being the products of any single factor, result from complex interactions between the child and his environment. The vital issue is not how heredity and environment are to be fractionated in the analysis of behavior, but precisely how the two interrelate and simultaneously influence the development of the individual . The clinician cannot possibly diagnose and treat patients effectively in terms of the traditional "nature versus nurture" concept. Constitutional determinants of behavior are modified by the environment in which they operate, and in turn the environment does not have a uniform impact on genetically diverse individuals.

A child's hereditary endowment interacts with environmental stimuli to produce a distinctive pattern of behavior. Since each child responds selectively to aspects of the world around him in terms of his own specific organismic characteristics, a given set of environmental circumstances does not have uniform consequences. Children differ widely, for example, in their susceptibility to the same external stresses and pressures. They have varied responses to similar patterns of parental care. Youngsters of like cultural and social backgrounds may show striking differences in personality and direction of development.

To assess the effect of any experience on a child—weaning, toilet-training, the birth of a sibling, going to school, or watching movies or television—requires knowledge not only of the event, but simultaneously of the child's characteristic reactions. Not only does the child screen his environment, he also influences it. Thus, it is not alone the parents who shape the child, but the child who affects parental reactions.

The existence of marked individuality in the spontaneous and reactive behavior of newborn infants has long been recognized by pediatricians, baby-nurses and experienced parents. Yet until recently little systematic attention has been paid to the child's own characteristics as a reactive organism. It is true that Freud (1950) asserted that "Each individual ego is endowed from the beginning with its own peculiar dispositions and tendencies." Pavlov postulated the existence of congenitally determined types of nervous systems as basic to the course of development.

Nevertheless, the earliest period of human life has been the last to receive systematic study. This lag is understandable, since the investigator of infant development faces peculiarly difficult problems. For one thing, the period from birth to two years of age encompasses the most rapid growth process of the entire lifetime, whether in terms of physiology, neurology or psychology. Another obvious difficulty in the study of infants is the absence of language, which makes it impossible to conduct the motivational explorations that rely on verbal communication of attitudes, feelings and purposes.

In recent years, however, an increasing number of studies have contributed to our understanding of the beginning phases of the child's growth and interrelationship with the world in which he is to live. These studies, based on direct observation of behavior, have revealed various abilities in infants at earlier ages than had been considered possible—for example, the capacity to follow objects visually, to discriminate between stimuli and to show pattern preferences. With the use of new techniques for measuring the infant's cognitive organization, as Charlesworth (1968) notes, modern research is challenging William James' famous assertion that "the baby, assailed by eyes, ears, nose, skin, and entrails at once, feels it all as one great blooming, buzzing confusion." Contrary to this traditional hypothesis, many recent studies have documented the fact that infants do not experience their world in identical terms. Instead, they show marked differences in various areas of behavior such as perceptual response, sensory threshold, autonomic response patterns, motility, and sleeping and feeding patterns.

The Role of Temperament

The individual child's temperament, or behavioral style, is a basic component of his development. The term "temperament" describes the characteristic tempo, rhythmicity, adaptability, energy expenditure, mood and attention-focus of a child, independent of the content of any specific behavior. The term refers to the *how* of behavior. It differs from ability, which is concerned with the *what* and *how well* of behaving. It is also to be distinguished from motivation, which seeks to account for *why* a person does what he is doing.

For example, two children may each throw a ball with accuracy, and have the same motives in so doing. Yet they may differ with respect to the intensity with which they act, the rate at which they move, the mood they express, their readiness to shift to a new activity, and the ease with which they will approach a new toy, situation or playmate.

Temperament is not immutable. Like any other characteristic of the organism, its features can undergo a developmental course that will be significantly affected by environmental circumstances.

To study the role of temperament in development, my colleagues (Thomas and Birch) and I undertook, in the mid-1950's, the New York Longitudinal Study of 136 children. The findings of this study are set forth in two volumes: *Behavioral Individuality in Early Childhood* (1963) and *Temperament and Behavior Disorders in Children* (1968). Since the children were studied from early life onward, and both their temperaments and environments were repeatedly assessed, it was possible to investigate two issues of importance for child psychiatry: (1) the manner in which temperamental patterns influence the likelihood that a behavior disorder will develop; and (2) the emergence of behavioral disturbance, together with the factors contributing to symptom formation and evolution.

Of the children in the study sample, 42 developed behavioral disturbances of various types and varying degrees of severity and duration. In each case the disturbance could be traced to a maladaptive interaction between a child with a particular temperamental pattern and significant features of his environment. It became clear that what constitutes a stressful situation or demand for a child depends as much upon the youngster's own temperament as upon the objective features of his environment. The success of any given set of child-care practices, therefore, depends on its suitability to the child, and no single set of rules will be optimal for all children.

The individual behavioral style of each child from the age of two to three months onward can be observed in terms of nine categories of reactivity:

1. *Activity level:* The motor component in a child's functioning, and the diurnal proportion of active and inactive periods.

2. *Rhythmicity:* The regularity and predictability of such functions as hunger, feeding pattern, elimination, and sleep-wake cycle.

3. *Approach or withdrawal:* The nature of the child's response to a new food, object, or person.

4. *Adaptability:* The speed and ease with which current behavior can be modified in response to altered environmental structuring.

5. *Intensity of reaction:* The energy level of response, irrespective of its quality or direction.

6. *Threshold of responsiveness:* The intensity level of stimulation required to evoke a discernible response to sensory stimuli, environmental objects, and social contacts.

7. *Quality of mood:* The amount of pleasant, joyful, or friendly behavior as contrasted with unpleasant, unfriendly behavior or crying.

8. *Distractibility:* The effectiveness of extraneous environmental stimuli in interfering with or in altering the direction of the ongoing behavior.

9. *Attention span and persistence:* The length of time a particular activity is pursued, and the continuation of an activity in the face of obstacles to maintaining the activity direction.

In general, the features of behavioral individuality that are identifiable in early infancy continue to characterize the child from year to year in his development. Though each child shows a range of behavior reactions in different situations and at different times, he can be identified by the preponderant mode of his reactions for each of the nine categories. The temperamental characteristics may be classified into a number of "constellations"—that is, specific patterns or clusters of the categories.

The temperamental constellation that characterizes the largest single group of children in the New York Study includes regularity of biologic function, adaptability to change, predominantly positive responses to new stimuli, a preponderance of positive mood, and reactions of mild or moderate intensity. This temperamental pattern defines "the easy child," who develops regular sleeping and feeding habits, and is easily able to adjust to new routines, new foods or a new school. He is usually able to handle frustration without becoming markedly distressed, and can comply smoothly and without tension with consistent parental demands.

As a group, the easy children develop proportionately fewer behavior problems than any other. But their very ease of adaptability may in certain circumstances be the basis for disturbance. Typically this occurs when behavior learned at home is not congruent with the norms of the peer group or the demands of the school situation. For the easy child, severe dissonance between the expectations and requirements of the intrafamilial and extrafamilial environments appears to be the most prominent source of stress resulting in psychologic disturbance.

The temperamental cluster that involves the highest risk of developing a behavior problem combines a set of characteristics at the other extreme: irregularity of biologic function, nonadaptability to change, predominantly negative responses to new stimuli, intense reactions and nondistractibility. The "difficult child" is not easy to feed, bathe, dress or put to sleep. His initial response to new foods, places or activities is characteristically negative, and the time required for adjustment prolonged. He typically reacts to frustration with loud crying or violent tantrums.

The specific sources of stress for the difficult child are the demands for socialization, that is, for altering spontaneous responses and patterns in conformity with the standards of the family, school or peer group. Demands for socialization tend to intensify stress to the point of symptom formation when they are made in an inconsistent, impatient or punitive manner.

There is no indication that parents of difficult children are essentially different from other parents or that they are in any way responsible for their children's temperamental characteristics. What does emerge is that parental attitudes and practices that are effective with most children are sometimes not adequate to promote smooth development and adaptation with a minimum of stress in the difficult children. All too often, however, parents react to the difficulties involved in handling such a child with resentment, guilt or a feeling of helplessness—with the result that a vicious circle is formed.

A third temperamental type is defined by a combination of negative, though mildly intense, initial responses to new situations, with gradual adaptation after repeated contact with the stimulus. The "slow-to-warm-up" children retreat from the new with either quiet withdrawal or mild trantrums, followed by adaptation when familiarity has been attained. Particularly stressful for such a child is parental insistence on an immediately positive response to a new food or a group of strange children. Pressure for quick adaptation typically intensifies the child's tendency to withdraw and may initiate a maladaptive child-environment interaction. If, on the other hand, slow adaptation is recognized as a part of the child's normal temperamental style and he is given patient encouragement, the child's ultimate response is usually one of positive interest and involvement.

These findings indicate that theories currently directing the diagnostic process in clinical child psychiatry are in need of restructuring. Much of the behavior that is considered solely in terms of the widely accepted concepts of anxiety, psychodynamic defenses and intrapsychic conflict can more parsimoniously be understood as the product of a maladaptive temperament-environment interaction. Anxiety, when it occurs, does not necessarily operate as a basic factor preceding the development of the problem behavior, but may derive secondarily from the stressful character of the maladaptive interactional process and the problem behavior.

The effectiveness of any therapeutic approach depends upon the accuracy with which the causes of disturbed behavior are diagnosed. For a sound evaluation, the clinician requires detailed data on the temperamental characteristics of the child. For example, an infant whose sleep is frequently interrupted by loud crying may be responding with anxiety to a hostile and rejecting mother; on the other hand, if he is a difficult child, this behavior may be a normal expression of his temperamental characteristics of biologic irregularity, negative mood and intensity of response. The accuracy of the differential diagnosis will depend on an assessment of both the mother's *and* the child's characteristics. Similarly, a child who is doing poorly in a permissive school setting may be resisting the academic pressuring of manipulative parents; but his underachievement may also be due to his distractibility and short attention span.

Much of current theory in child psychiatry assumes that a child's behavior is directly and exclusively related to maternal attitudes and practices, and therapy tends to focus on the supposedly noxious influences of the mother on the child. But parental influences must be evaluated with reference to the child's own characteristics. While a mother's guilt and anxiety may be evidence of a neurosis, they may also be a response to the problems involved in handling a very difficult child. Parental influences must be considered in terms of a specific child-environment interaction. To do so, temperament must be given the same systematic attention that is now devoted to maternal and other environmental factors.

Mastery and Learning

The infant advances toward mature behavior by mastering his environment with the use of the organs with which he is endowed. Whether one refers to this process as "mastery" or "learning," the normal infant gradually progresses from a state in which he is unable to perform a particular task to a state in which it is successfully accomplished. Then he proceeds in the same way to master the next task confronting him.

The style of learning varies from infant to infant but is consistent for any one child. By deliberately structuring a learning situation in accordance with the child's style of learning, an adult familiar with the youngster may facilitate his mastery of situations. Such mastery may be retarded if the adult inflexibly follows a set of rules.

Modes of learning are innumerable. One child will look around for praise repeatedly during hours of practice spent in putting one foot in front of another as he goes back and forth between chair and table. Another will make his initial attempts to walk only when he is alone. Still another will hold on to chairs or seem to cherish the illusion that he is being supported by push-toys long after it is clear to the observer that the youngster has mastered a new skill and no longer needs physical help in walking. Similarly, one baby who drops a doll out of her carriage will patiently yank at its string while cheerfully calling to some passerby to help her, whereas another child in the same situation will cry in rage and make no attempt to retrieve the doll.

The tactics used by parents or others in child rearing will have different behavioral results depending on the nature of the child to whom they are applied. Too often, however, we talk in generalities, referring to an optimum age for weaning or for instituting toilet-training. Yet it is logical, for example, to expect that the baby who established a regular rhythm in elimination at an early age will be toilet-trained through simple conditioning, while one with an irregular pattern may not be able to achieve full control of his sphincter until he is old enough to approach the task consciously and deliberately.

It is certainly true that such factors as maternal overprotection or rejection, or a punitive approach by the father, have been found to be associated with disturbances in the development of a child's learning or mastery. But so much has been written about parent-child hostility and the child's resentment of dependency that one is apt to get the impression that the rearing of a child is always a traumatic process. Many a well-read mother is left with only one hope—that she will not show up too badly in her child's analysis when he becomes a maladjusted adult. The process of socialization, which ought to be experienced as a cooperative endeavor in which parent and child, as partners, take genuine pride in each of the child's new achievements, is all too often represented as a primarily painful conflict engendering mutual resentment and hostility between parent and child.

As a result, many parents try to operate on the theory that they must not frustrate a child or do anything that will create conflict for him. In actuality, neither frustration nor conflict is in itself destructive. The child who is never frustrated, whose conflicts are resolved for him by eliminating or easing those factors that militate against the spontaneous expression and satisfactions of his desires, becomes well-adjusted only to an extremely artificial set of circumstances. When such a youngster approaches the later stages of socialization which his parents do not control, as on entering school, he will lack the kind of experience that would help him to know how to respond to each new situation. Many behavior disorders appear at this point.

Human growth is stimulated by conflict. A child would have little incentive to learn how to speak if his inability to express a wish did not interfere with its being granted. Were it not for the desire to join his peers, the youngster would not learn how to take his place in a peer group, to share, to assert himself, and to deal with swift and dramatic changes in "junior" human relations. Much as the toddler, who falls when he is so close to the ground that he cannot hurt himself, learns to pick himself up, the child learns how to master frustration and conflict by dealing with them before they have acquired negative social meanings. The youngster who is unable to hold the continuous and undivided attention of his mother gains socially from learning to master this frustration constructively.

Learning to get along with a sibling is about the best preparation a child can have for establishing good human relations with his peers. A youngster may develop a concept of cooperative behavior if he comes to understand that his parents are giving him a fair share of their attention, and that they will not accede to his demands for more because this would deprive a sibling of his share of attention. The readiness of children for new experiences and new demands cannot be mechanically scheduled. There is a fairly wide range of ages for each successful effort to control behavior. In this respect, too, individual differences in physiology, maturation and temperament play an important part.

Social and Cultural Influences

It has already been noted that a child with a behavior problem must be studied in the light of his preproblem behavior, not in comparison with some stereotype of what is considered to be "normal" behavior. Similarly, he must be studied within the frame of reference of his particular environment. His behavior must be assessed not in accordance with arbitrary criteria, which all too often are based on what is acceptable in the culture of the therapist, but rather with full awareness of the standards that prevail in the child's culture. This point cannot be too strongly emphasized.

A child growing up in the slums of a large city is likely to develop different behavior patterns from those of one raised in an affluent suburb of the same city. On the other hand, a child growing up in a university town in California will be subjected to many of the same influences that affect one growing up in a New England university community. In evaluating a child's behavior, it is essential to take into account his socioeconomic and cultural identification. One must know whether the behavior corresponds to or deviates from the adaptation of his group.

Thus the reactions of a Negro child living in the inner city may appear "pathologic" to an uninformed observer although these reactions may in fact be an expression of protective behavior that is appropriate. While the psychiatrist cannot ordinarily go and live with a child's family in order to have a proper assessment of his behavior, he should at least strive to overcome the limitations of his own socioeconomic perspective.

As Coles (1967) has pointed out in *Children of Crisis,* youngsters in a minority group subject to discrimination have a definite concept of "in" people and "out" people. Their behavior with strangers or authorities may give an impression of excessive suspiciousness and other "abnormal" behaviors that are not actually expressions of their character structures or their typical ways of acting. Their suspiciousness is rational in terms of their group's experience. "The relationship between the emerging personality pattern and the social stresses is not of course a simple and direct one," as Kenneth Clark (1955) notes. "Students of personality are forced to recognize that the complexity of personality and society makes it difficult to isolate any one factor of a complex society and demonstrate unequivocally the effect of this single factor upon the whole personality of an individual. Nevertheless, the evidence from social-science research, from general observations, from clinical material, and from theoretical analyses consistently indicates that the personality pattern of minority-group individuals is influenced by the fact of their minority status."

It is often assumed that "disadvantaged" children are to be identified only in terms of the negative influences that the environment exerts on their development. This is a serious misconception. While it is, of course, true that a background of poverty, disease and poor schooling has an adverse and sometimes disastrous effect, it does not automatically follow that children who come from such a handicapping environment are emotionally or intellectually blighted. The psychologic hazards and educational penalties are undeniable. But psychiatrists are increasingly impressed with the strengths as well as the vulnerabilities of the "disadvantaged" child. Recent studies, many of them related to school desegregation, have noted not merely the negative impact of deprivation but also the resilience, toughness and resourcefulness shown by many such children.

Cultural influences are not automatically absorbed by the child with the air he breathes. They are transmitted to him primarily by other people in the course of the interpersonal relationships in which he is involved. These relationships, then, must also be understood by the therapist as a necessary and important factor in the child's cultural environment.

The most fundamental of the child's interpersonal connections are those with his parents, or parent substitutes. As the child grows older, his relationships with his siblings and peers bulk large. His teachers and other adults with whom he has contact also help to form his attitudes. Even people with whom he has no direct physical contact, such as sports heroes or TV or movie idols, often play a great part in fashioning the child's personality.

Clearly, the attitudes of parents or parent substitutes toward the young child are an especially vital influence in shaping his behavior. These attitudes, however, are not those of abstract mother or father figures existing in a vacuum. Parents are themselves continually affected by cultural forces. Parent attitudes toward their children vary in respect to cultural background, personality make-up, economic status, and the particular pediatric and psychologic theories that are currently fashionable.

The trend today, for example, is for the father to play a caretaker role to a greater extent than in the past. Again, in middle-class families in the United States, the present focus is on satisfying the child's needs in infancy and early childhood, and the household tends to be child-centered. On the other hand, in the lower economic groups, with larger families and children more closely spaced, there is perforce less concentration on satisfying each expressed need of an individual child. The older siblings are expected to perform chores and take some responsibility for the care of the younger children. Thus the parent-child relationship is not an unchanging thing in different periods and in different social groups.

Nor do extrafamilial and intrafamilial factors operate in isolation from each other. In some cases extrafamilial forces tend to intensify parental influence; in others, they may modify or attenuate it; and in still other instances, they may produce consequences for a child's development that are different from but harmonious with those influenced by parental functioning. For example, a parent may be fostering negativistic tendencies in a slowly adaptive child by insisting on quick adaptations to new situations that are difficult for the youngster to make. If the nursery school teacher makes similar demands, the influences encouraging negativistic trends will be intensified. But if she allows the child to adapt at his own pace, the negativistic tendencies may at least in part be modified. Thus it can never be assumed that the direction and intensity of a child's reaction to parental influence occur in isolation or necessarily continue unchanged as he grows older.

One should keep in mind that grandparents, aunts, uncles, cousins and other relatives may be members of the household or frequent visitors, and that extremely strong positive or negative attachments can spring up between them and the child. Interaction with these family figures may create identifications, antagonisms or ambivalences in the child; and these patterns of response may be as important determinants of his behavior as the interrelationships within the primary family group.

Influence of Peer Groups

The psychiatrist can scarcely understand a given child's behavior unless he has some knowledge of the youngster's peers. At a very early age, the child moves out into a society that no longer consists only of his family. He becomes increasingly aware of the behavior of other children, and this acts as a stimulant for further development of his own behavior. The peer group becomes an effective force in lessening the child's dependency on the mother.

The child observes and imitates. Not infrequently he begins his toilet training by copying an older brother or sister or some child of his own age who has been toilet trained. It is not unusual to have a child who had been content to eat in the high chair insist on taking his place at the table in imitation of another child. The stimulus for going to school alone, crossing the street by himself, or at a later age for making his first trip on a bus or train by himself, often comes when the child observes that his behavior is out of keeping with that of other children whom he admires. Perhaps the most exquisite expression of the influence of the peer group is in adolescence, at which time the youngster can sometimes be stimulated dramatically to healthier and more mature behavior or the converse.

The changing mores in peer groups are sometimes difficult for the psychiatrist to keep in touch with, but try he must. For example, in the current "sexual revolution" among adolescents, a whole new set of moral values is being developed. The "revolution" is largely determined by the fact that girls can be free of the fear of pregnancy accompanying sexual experimentation. Members of an older generation, which inevitably includes the psychiatrist and the youngster's parents, find it hard to detach their own moral views and background from the question of what makes for deep and sincere relationships. The fact is that most youngsters are very much concerned with the question of how much sexual "freedom" is consistent with the ideal of mature love. Their behavior can be evaluated only if one understands that their concepts are strongly influenced by the sexual practices in their peer groups.

Currently, the hippie or flower-child movement is the subject of much discussion. When an adolescent is brought to psychiatric attention because of parental disapproval of his way of life, one must have some awareness of what the current adolescent behavior is with regard to the complaints. This does not mean that if the child's behavior is in complete agreement with a fad this makes it normal. If one had a whole population of children who were undernourished, one would not call an individual child's undernourishment normal; it may be that a whole group had abnormal nutrition. In the same way, the dancing manias of the middle ages, even though they swept whole populations, did not constitute normal behavior.

Nevertheless, it is important to know whether a child's behavior is out of keeping not only with his parents' but also the peer group's mores. The behavior may reflect a fad rather than an idiosyncratic departure. A fad may attract youngsters whose basic psychologic organization is normal. It may also be the framework on which major psychopathology is expressed.

Basically normal adolescents may experiment with drugs and display startlingly offbeat modes of personal grooming that reflect the current style of a peer group. On the other hand, the same ways of life may be taken up by youngsters who are psychologically disturbed. A chronicle of drugs taken or of strange living patterns will not itself reveal what is essentially normal or abnormal.

Conflict of Cultures

A conflict between two sets of cultural attitudes may generate behavioral problems. This occurs when a child is suddenly taken out of one environment and placed in another, or when he encounters in his extrafamilial relationships a completely different set of standards from those he has known in his own family group.

Let us, for example, look at the case of an eleven year old Puerto Rican boy referred for treatment as a behavior problem by school authorities in New York City. He was described as chronically late in arriving at school, disruptive in class, and generally involved in any classroom disturbance. In addition, the complaint was made that he dressed negligently, with no sense of decorum. Projective tests showed indications of belligerence and hostility in his personality. The school authorities considered the boy's family to be indifferent to his problem.

The boy himself, in an interview with the therapist, showed a cooperative attitude and declared that he liked New York (he had come from Puerto Rico with his family only a year before) and could not understand why he was having trouble. The parents, when interviewed, also insisted that their son was a good boy and no problem at home.

Confronted with such a situation, with contradictory reports from different sources, a psychiatrist who was not oriented to a consideration of cultural influences might be immobilized by not knowing where to start. Or he might concentrate on building a good relationship with the child and thereupon brush away the reports of the child's problems as nonsense. On the other hand, a merely superficial acceptance of the importance of cultural forces might lead the therapist to see this as simply "another case" of a Puerto Rican boy unable to adjust to the big city.

An intensive and detailed study of the social and cultural factors involved, however, revealed a number of significant facts. The boy had grown up in an impoverished rural area in Puerto Rico, where a shortage of qualified teachers, and other problems, made for sporadic schooling. The boy had no concept of the need for regular and punctual school attendance, and had no orientation to the scheduled completion of school assignments. The poverty of the area was such that the question of wearing special clothes to school never came up.

In his new life in New York, this background as well as his ignorance of English made school a bewildering experience to him. The teacher criticized him, and his schoolmates taunted him, for reasons his experience had not fitted him to understand. His adjustment to his new life was further delayed by the fact that his parents, fearful of his becoming involved with a street gang, forbade him to play outside. As a further factor in the boy's confusion, the relationships in his own family had shifted markedly. The father, unable to find regular work in New York, was now at home much of the time, while the mother, a skilled seamstress, took on a full-time job.

A knowledge of all these specific factors enabled the therapist to put into proper perspective the seemingly variant reports of school authorities and parents, to evaluate properly the boy's own attitudes and conflicts, and to begin to work out a helpful approach to his problems.

Behavior problems sometimes arise because the child comes into conflict with the cultural standards of his parents. Such conflicts are likely to occur in the United States because cultural groupings are not static. The second generation American child of immigrant parents is less affected by his family's culture than were his parents. Class culture is particularly mobile, since it is so closely related to economic position and educational status, and these, as is well known, change rapidly in this country from generation to generation.

The child may come from a racial group in which the patriarchal family is the accepted pattern and the father is the unquestioned authority figure. Any deviation from complete acceptance of this pattern by the child is likely to be considered delinquent behavior by the parents. Action by the child that in another culture might be considered the normal groping toward independence may be regarded in this culture as behavior meriting drastic punishment. This way of handling the child may set up a chain reaction going from rebellion to antisocial acts.

All these considerations emphasize that the therapist, in treating a behavior problem, must analyze the child's environment for mores which have persisted and those which have been modified or diffused by impact with other cultures. It is of paramount importance to understand how and to what extent the child's behavior deviates from the cultural pattern of his family and his group, since it is this deviation that is significant rather than the deviation from some hypothetic optimum way of behaving.

Even where there is no obvious shift in cultural patterns between the parents' generation and the child's generation, culturally determined parental attitudes may play a major role in the development of real or apparent behavior problems in the child. The attitudes of parents toward their children may be direct reflections or distorted reflections of the culture in which they were reared. The parent may slavishly follow or violently reject the mores of his own culture. Between these extremes of espousal and rejection are many gradations of attitude.

If the male is preeminently important in the parents' culture, this attitude is likely to show up in how the male or female infant is handled; a boy will be favored, often to the detriment of his sisters.

Similarly, the child will be esteemed according to the extent to which he manifests certain qualities that have prestige in the parents' culture or social group, such as belligerency, gregariousness, intellectual attainments or conventional good looks. Conversely, of course, the child will be a disappointment to the parents insofar as he does not show the traits that are valued.

Such cultural patterns influence the parents in terms of their own personalities, their own areas of strength and weakness, their personality needs, hopes, fears and insecurities, and their attitudes about what is desirable and enjoyable in life. For example, the mother who was herself a tomboy and as a child suffered from being continuously told to behave "like a little lady," may take great pleasure in relating to a physically active, outgoing son or daughter. On the other hand, if her youngster is quiet and retiring, she may be resentful, see personality problems where none exist, and possibly even create behavior disorders by her antagonism toward the child. In either case, she is reacting not to the child, but in a complex way to the unresolved confusions and conflicts that she herself had as a child. To cite another example, the father who is a boxing fan and perhaps enjoys boxing himself is all too often unable to comprehend that a quiet, unaggressive son should be allowed to develop along the lines that are in keeping with his own personality. The father prods the boy into being aggressive, urges him to "stand up and fight," and the boy—by his very nature doomed to failure in this role—responds with fear in all his peer relationships.

The parent, mouthing the conventionally correct middle-class ideas, may say, "I don't care whether or not my child is smart. All I want is for him to be happy." Actually, if the parent is somewhat insecure about his own intellectual competence or if his culture places great emphasis on intellectual achievements, he will be disappointed if his offspring shows below-average or only average intelligence. Pressure is put on the child to attain goals that are beyond his capacity. This attitude shows up particularly clearly when the child is being helped with homework. Instead of patiently suggesting a good approach to a problem, the parent is irritable and critical, thus increasing the child's insecurity and lack of self-confidence.

Parental attitudes, however, are only one factor in the range of environmental influences. They must be assessed in conjunction with all the other forces that impinge on the growing child.

34 INTRODUCTION TO CHILD PSYCHIATRY

SELECTED REFERENCES

Baldwin, A. L.: *Theories of Child Development.* New York, Wiley, 1967.

Bowlby, J.: *Maternal Care and Mental Health.* Geneva, World Health Organization, 1951.

Bridger, W. H.: Sensory discrimination and autonomic function in the newborn. *J. Amer. Acad. Child Psychiat.* 1:67-82, 1962.

Charlesworth, W. R.: Cognition in infancy: where do we stand in the mid-sixties? *Merrill-Palmer Quarterly* 14:25-46, 1968.

Chess, S., Clark, K. B., and Thomas, A.: The importance of cultural evaluation in psychiatric diagnosis and treatment. *Psychiatric Quarterly* 27:102-114, 1953.

Chess, S., Thomas, A., and Birch, H. G.: *Your Child Is A Person.* New York, Viking, 1965.

Clark, K. B.: *Prejudice and Your Child.* Boston, Beacon Press, 1955.

Coles, R.: *Children of Crisis.* Boston, Little, Brown, 1967.

Erikson, E. H.: *Childhood and Society.* New York, W. W. Norton, 1950.

Freud, A.: *The Ego and Mechanisms of Defense.* London, Hogarth Press, 1948.

Freud, S.: *Collected Papers,* Vols. I-V. London, Hogarth Press, 1924-1953.

Freud, S.: Analysis terminable and interminable. *Collected Papers,* Vol. 5. London, Hogarth Press, 1950.

Fromm, E.: *The Sane Society.* New York, Rinehart & Co., 1955.

Gesell, A., and Ilg, F. L.: *Infant and Child in the Culture of Today.* New York, Harper and Brothers, 1943.

Hollingshead, A., and Redlich, F.: *Social Class and Mental Illness.* New York, Wiley, 1958.

Kardiner, A.: *The Psychological Frontiers of Society.* New York, Columbia University Press, 1945.

Kretschmer, E.: *Physique and Character.* London, Kegan Paul, 1925.

Levy, D.: *Maternal Overprotection.* New York, Columbia University Press, 1943.

Murphy, L. B.: *The Widening World of Childhood.* New York, Basic Books, 1962.

Papousek, H.: Conditioning during early postnatal development. *In* Brackbill, Y., and Thompson, G. (Eds.): *Behavior in Infancy and Early Childhood.* New York, The Free Press, 1967.

Pavlov, I. P.: *Conditioned Reflexes.* Trans. G. V. Anrep. London, Oxford University Press, 1927.

Piaget, J.: *The Language and Thought of the Child.* 3rd edition. New York, Humanities Press, 1959.

Ribble, M.: *The Rights of Infants.* New York, Columbia University Press, 1943.

Sears, R. R., Maccoby, E. E., and Levin, H.: *Patterns of Child Rearing.* Evanston, Ill., Peterson, 1957.

Sheldon, W. H.: *Varieties of Human Physique.* New York, Harper and Brothers, 1940.

Thomas, A., Birch, H. G., Chess, S., Hertzig, M. E., and Korn, S.: *Behavioral Individuality in Early Childhood.* New York, New York University Press, 1963.

Thomas, A., Chess, S., and Birch, H. G.: *Temperament and Behavior Disorders in Children.* New York, New York University Press, 1968.

Watson, J. B.: *Behaviorism.* London, Kegan Paul, 1925.

3. Genetic Factors in Behavior

RECENT ADVANCES in biochemical genetics and microscopy have had a profound impact on child psychiatry as on other branches of medicine. Psychiatrists have long known that genetically transmitted defects may cause mental retardation. Now there is a growing body of evidence that a number of behavior aberrations, whether or not accompanied by mental deficiency, are also determined by hereditary factors. An awareness of genetic issues has therefore become essential for the child psychiatrist.

The ability to identify inborn metabolic defects can be crucial for differential diagnosis. For example, the behavioral picture of phenylketonuria may resemble certain features of other syndromes, including childhood schizophrenia. The disease may manifest itself in psychotic behavior, mental retardation or seizures, as well as in unusually light pigmentation and eczema; the symptoms may be present in various combinations. Thanks to the widespread testing for phenylketonuria, this disorder has been identified in some children who might previously have been treated for some other illness.

Another example of a disease that has been clarified by genetic study is Down's syndrome, also referred to as Langdon-Down disease or mongolism. The clinical characteristics of this disease include a typical facial configuration: wide-spaced eyes, flattened bridge of the nose, an epicanthal fold at the inner corner of the eye, small mouth and a large protruding tongue. There are also abnormalities of the hand, and congenital heart defects are often found. In the past, this disease was attributed to purely environmental influences such as maternal intercurrent infection during the first trimester. Today we know that Down's syndrome is caused by a definable and even photographable chromosomal defect.

But genetic factors cannot be considered in isolation, since the organism is in continuous interaction with its environment. As J. D. Rainer (1967) notes, "There are many pathways from identical genetic structures to later expression of behavioral traits, and minor shifts of interaction at crucial points may lead to wide divergence in phenotypes."

The expression of a hereditary defect can be significantly modified by environmental influences. In emphasizing this fact, the modern geneticist is perhaps the strongest environmentalist. Specific circumstances, he recognizes, may bring to the fore a genetic fault that in another setting would not be operative and therefore not even recognized as a fault. For example, an individual who has inherited vulnerability to a given allergen will not be "allergic" if the offending substance is not present in his environment. Some investigators have suggested that the defect in phenylketonuria is not operative unless certain amino acids are present in the diet.

Similarly, the potential behavioral effects of a genetic fault may be modifiable through environmental manipulation. To recognize the hereditary basis of a behavioral disorder, therefore, is not to become a defeatist. On the contrary, it is the signal for mobilizing all available resources for limiting the negative consequences of the defect. A correct diagnosis of the inborn fault may be the precondition for appropriate handling of the child.

As Down's syndrome, phenylketonuria and other genetically determined developmental abnormalities have come under study, the picture has become less simple than was initially believed. Down's syndrome does not have a unitary genetic cause; there are three known patterns of chromosomal fault. Similarly, the metabolic defect in phenylketonuria does not always seem to have a continuous effect. Phenylketones may appear in the urine at some periods and not at others. Defective children with phenylketonuria are sometimes found to have sibs who also have this condition but do not have definable defects of intellect or behavior.

An understanding of such problems enables the psychiatrist to counsel parents, who, having had one child that was born defective, want to know if it would be advisable for them to have another child. While the psychiatrist is not expected to be an expert in this field, he must be sufficiently acquainted with the problem to recognize the circumstances that require genetic investigation and counseling by a specialist.

Problems of Transmission

The new advances in genetics, while adding immeasurably to our understanding of heredity, have been built upon the foundation of classic genetics. In some cases, questions of hereditary transmission can be understood in purely Mendelian terms.

Phenylketonuria, for example, is currently considered to be due to a single autosomal inheritance of a faulty chromosome which is recessive. This means that the parents are not phenylketonuric themselves, but are heterozygous carriers; that is, each has one defective chromosome paired with a nondefective chromosome, and their children have one in four possibilities of inheriting the defective chromosomes and hence having the active disorder. The chromosomal error affects the production of phenylalanine hydroxylase, the enzyme that oxidizes phenylalanine to tyrosine. There is either insufficient production of the enzyme or a failure to produce it at all. As a result of the abnormal metabolism, phenylpyruvic acid is excreted and the blood contains large amounts of phenylalanine.

Heterozygous carriers, while symptom-free, have a reduced enzyme level that can be detected by a phenylalanine-tolerance test (the Guthrie test). Ever since the importance of this syndrome has been established, the Guthrie test has been done on a mass scale. Some states require that the test be done on all newborn infants. The incidence of the disease, formerly considered to be 1 in 25,000 births, is now estimated as 1 in 10,000 births.

In other diseases, such as Down's syndrome, the study of hereditary transmission has required a modification of classic genetics. In Down's syndrome, as Lejeune (1964) was the first to point out, a genetic abnormality results from nondisjunction of either chromosome 21 or 22. As a result, the full chromosomal material, instead of half, goes to the daughter cell. If this abnormal cell is fertilized, the zygote has 47 rather than the normal 46 chromosomes. This trisomy is typically found in older mothers.

The concordance rate in one-egg twins is close to 100 percent. The risk of having a child with Down's syndrome is one in fifty for mothers over age 45. However, if a mother in this age group has had one child with Down's syndrome due to trisomy, the risk of having a second defective child is no greater than for other mothers in the same age group.

A mosaic pattern in the occurrence of Down's syndrome has also been described. In this pattern, the extra chromosome is lost through disjunction in a very early cell division; two cell lines occur in the individual, who then has some cells with 46 and some with

47 chromosomes. Patients with the mosaic pattern tend to have intermediate symptomatology.

Still another type of Down's syndrome is due to translocation; that is, the extra chromosomal material from 21 or 22 attaches to the chromosome of another group. While the total chromosomal count is the normal 46, the risk in a carrier parent is one in three that the children will have Down's syndrome. A defective child with this type of inheritance is likely to be of young parents.

Clearly, then, the fact that a family has one child with Down's syndrome is not in itself a guide to the degree of risk that a second child will be born defective. Without genetic investigation, it would not be possible to give the parents an accurate assessment of the risk.

Sex-Linked Behavioral Deviations

In medicine, the best known sex-linked disorder is hemophilia, which in its classic form is a disease of males but transmitted by females. This phenomenon has certain counterparts in psychiatry. Anomalies in the X and Y chromosomes are involved in Turner's syndrome and a number of other clinical conditions that have behavioral implications.

Crucial for this area of study is the fact that in 1949 Barr found that when the buccal mucosal cells of normal females were stained according to his procedure, 30 to 60 per cent showed a dark mass near the cell membrane. This probably represents one of the two X chromosomes, the one that is inactive. In males there should be no Barr bodies. In 1954 further work showed that the presence of a drumstick-like appendage to one of the lobes of the polymorphonuclear leukocytes could distinguish between chromosomal maleness or femaleness.

In Turner's syndrome, which involves incomplete sexual development in females, there is a total of only 45 chromosomes, one of the X chromosomes being absent. Since no Barr body is found in the XO female, it is assumed that the normally inactive X has not been transmitted because of nondisjunction. The syndrome appears in 1 in 3,000 female births. Typically, the morphology is that of a short female with infantile genitalia, the gonads consisting only of connective tissue.

Klinefelter's syndrome occurs in males who have an extra X chromosome, giving a total of 47 chromosomes. The Barr body is present in the XXY abnormality, which appears in 1 of every 350 male births. In this syndrome there are atrophic testes, sterility, gynecomastia and mental retardation.

A syndrome in which there are three X chromosomes results in sexual infantility and amenorrhea despite the superabundance of female chromosomal material. Some investigators have noted a high incidence of aggressive criminality among XYY males.

In addition to chromosomal studies, there are other modes of genetic investigation that may throw light on behavioral disorders. These techniques include the pedigree survey, census analysis, research into studies of familial risk as compared with risk expectancy in the general population, and twin studies.

Chromosomal Breaks

Of great interest to the child psychiatrist is the rapidly growing body of research dealing with chromosomal breaks. The following is a brief summary of current knowledge about this phenomenon and its consequences.

Chromosomal breaks can be caused by ionizing radiation, viruses or drugs. They may result in a rearrangement of chromosomal material or in missing or extra material.

Unstable aberrations may last only for two or three cell divisions and then disappear. Ninety-five per cent of chromosomal breaks, such as those occurring after an acute viral infection, heal normally and do not constitute any permanent genetic damage. It is the stable aberrations, lasting for many years, that are of concern.

The aberrations are of three types:

1. A chromatid break is found in a single arm of the chromosome in the process of division. Restitution of the break is possible.

2. A chromatid gap is not a real discontinuity in the chromosomal substance. It tends to heal and does not cause abnormalities.

3. A chromosomal (or isochromatid) break occurs in the same place on both arms of the chromosome. The telomere, or end of the chromosome, is normally not "sticky"; however, when a break occurs, the newly created ends are sticky and can join in various ways, thus producing chromosomal rearrangement, the most dangerous form of aberration. The rearrangements include dicentric forms with two centromeres, ring chromosomes, and various types of translo-

cations that give chromosomes the shape of a cross with three points or other abnormal shapes.

The crucial issue for genetic transmission is whether such rearrangements are represented in the final division of the germ cell. If two homologous chromosomes break and join, the egg or sperm will get two of the four elements instead of one. Depending on these elements, the germ cell will either be normal or homozygous for a whole block of genes. There are other possibilities of rearrangement: two nonhomologous chromosomes may break and join, or more than two chromosomes may be involved.

Normally, an individual carries from four to ten dangerous or lethal recessive genes, which will come to notice only if the mate also carries one of these genes; both parents must contribute the recessive gene to the fertilized egg. But a chromosomal break that gives a daughter cell two homozygous dangerous genes requires only one parent to donate the recessive defect.

In actual practice, most drugs that cause chromosomal breaks are used in treating cancer in either terminal patients or those who are beyond the reproductive age. However, if such drugs are used in patients who survive and are within reproductive age, there could be danger to the offspring. With lethal or sufficiently dangerous genes, the fetus will not survive, but if the abnormal genes do not cause uterine death a malformed child may be born. It is also possible that a child carrying balanced translocations would be the carrier of a new abnormality, although he himself would be normal.

This problem has become an issue for the psychiatrist because he may be called upon to treat young people who are using a variety of drugs, including LSD, which have been reported to produce chromosomal breaks. While the possible genetic consequences of such drugs have not yet been clearly established, the psychiatrist must keep himself at least as well informed on current investigations as do his adolescent patients.

LSD studies have shown that the drug may increase the normal incidence of chromosomal breaks (about 3 per cent) by two or four times. Chromosomal studies of eighteen patients have been carried out by Drs. Cohen, Hirschhorn and Frosch (1967). The patients had taken LSD in varying dosages and with varying frequency. Chromosomal breaks and rearrangements were identified both during the period of active drug use and for at least six to eight months after the last use of LSD. In a few of the subjects the number of breaks was not much above the upper limits of normal, suggesting that there may be an individual susceptibility. There was no correlation between the degree of chromosomal breakage and the clinical evidence of adverse psychiatric effects, such as psychosis.

Three of the subjects were mothers who had taken LSD during pregnancy; one of these had two children and the others had one each. All of the four children showed chromosomal breaks and aberrant rearrangements that persisted. While the children appeared normal otherwise, the question to be asked is whether they are now carriers of abnormal genes.

Thus the genetic issue has invaded the area of diagnosis in younger children. It has stimulated new research into the etiology of behavioral and intellectual aberrations. In addition, the new findings about chromosomal breaks have raised the issue of helping youngsters understand that drug experimentation is not merely a matter of personal preference affecting only oneself, but may be harmful to a later generation.

SELECTED REFERENCES

Anderson, V. E.: Genetics in mental retardation. *In* Stevens, H. A., and Heber, R. (Eds.): *Mental Retardation.* Chicago, University of Chicago Press, 1964.

Beadle, G., and Beadle, M.: *The Language of Life.* New York, Doubleday, 1966.

Cohen, M. M., Hirschhorn, K., and Frosh, W. A.: In vivo and in vitro chromosonal damage induced by LSD-25. *New Eng. J. Med.* 277(20):1043-1049, 1967.

Gottesman, I. L.: Genetic aspects of intelligent behavior. *In* Ellis, N. R. (Ed.): *Handbook of Mental Deficiency.* New York, McGraw-Hill, 1963.

Kallmann, F. J. (Ed.): *Expanding Goals of Genetics in Psychiatry.* New York, Grune & Stratton, 1962.

Lejeune, J.: The 21-trisomy—current stage of chromosomal research. *In* Steinberg, A. G., and Bearn, A. G. (Eds.): *Progress in Medical Genetics.* New York, Grune & Stratton, 1964.

McClearn, G. E.: Behavioral genetics: An overview. *Merrill-Palmer Quart.* 14:9-24, 1968.

Rainer, J. D.: Genetics and psychiatry. *In* Freedman, A. M., and Kaplan, H. I. (Eds.): *Comprehensive Textbook of Psychiatry.* Baltimore, Williams & Wilkins, 1967.

4. The Presenting Problems

How WIDESPREAD are behavior disorders among children in the United States? Impressions, opinions, and hypotheses are plentiful, but it is impossible to answer the question accurately. Epidemiologists have made much less headway in assessing the prevalence of psychiatric disorders, either in adults or in children, than in estimating the incidence of physical disease.

The reasons for the uncertainty about the number of children in need of psychiatric care are manifold. Not only have relatively few prevalence surveys been completed, but even these have covered limited geographic areas. Moreover, no true statistical picture can be drawn from these studies, since they are based on different criteria of what constitutes psychiatric disorder. They have been conducted with different degrees of intensity. The most superficial surveys represent a compilation of the total cases reported by various kinds of institutions dealing with the mentally ill, while psychiatric examinations and other validating procedures mark the most intensive and scientifically conducted samplings. Some surveys, mechanically based on child admissions to state hospitals and child-care institutions, err by including all mentally retarded youngsters and even normal dependent children receiving custodial care. Such surveys fail to account for children receiving outpatient psychiatric treatment, either privately or in a clinic.

The degree of disturbance that leads physicians, hospitals, juvenile courts, school authorities and social workers to ticket a child as a behavior problem varies from area to area. Urban centers tend to focus on certain types of complaints that often receive little attention in rural districts; the reverse is also true. Even a parent's decision that his child needs help is largely influenced by the social patterns of his community. Judgment of the child's behavior as normal or deviant is usually based on a comparison with the behavior of other children of the same age in the area where he lives.

In large city schools, still another factor must be taken into account in evaluating the accuracy of statistics on children requiring psychiatric care. In many regions, children who need treatment are not recommended for it simply because there is a dearth of facilities. Teachers and principals tend to feel that there is no point in ticketing as behavior problems many children who need guidance, in view of the length of the waiting lists at diagnostic and treatment centers.

The Range of Problems

The range of behavior patterns that may constitute problem areas expands as the preschool child passes from one age period to the next. Reports of aberrant activity in an infant focus characteristically on sleep patterns, eating habits, hypermotility and the like. A complaint may concern a ten month old baby who rocks on hands and knees for hours at a time, or bangs his head against his crib. Another complaint may relate to an infant of fifteen months who refuses to ingest any solid food. A child of two who bites other children or a three year old who goes into prolonged tantrums or gives evidence of excessive frustration will arouse the concern of some parents. Others will complain that their youngster of five grabs the toys of his playmates and frequently hits them without any provocation.

As the child reaches school age and theoretically becomes capable of new types of functioning and of adjusting to new social situations, he may continue to manifest behavior more characteristic of the preschool child, in addition to conducting himself inappropriately in other respects. Any failure to achieve the more mature social conduct of which he is then deemed capable may worry his parents. Delay in sphincter control, which may have been tolerated at an earlier age, becomes a matter of great concern. Masturbation or sex play with other children may greatly alarm the parents. Aggressiveness, which seemed to be of minor import a few years earlier, may militate against the child's acceptance by his schoolmates. Shyness and emotional withdrawal also become more obvious at the age when he is expected to widen his circle of acquaintances. Learning difficulties begin to figure more prominently among the problems for which parents seek professional advice. Undue dependency which was not recognized when the child was younger may give rise to excessive demands for his teacher's attention; undetected anxiety

over separation from a parent may blossom into a phobia about going to school. Fears may become more pronounced and take the form
of apprehension over being involved in specific experiences such as
kidnapping, fire or burglary. Hyperactivity, which may not have
been ranked as a major problem before the child entered school,
may have to be investigated at a teacher's insistence.

As the child gets closer and closer to the relative independence of
adolescence, problems characteristic of the earlier stage may seem
to drop out altogether, but in reality often persist with changed
characteristics. The adolescent may become more effectively disruptive in manifesting a defiance of adult standards. Hence, a substantial number of preadolescents and adolescents are referred for
treatment because of their clashes with authority figures. Habitual
disputes between a parent and a negativistic youngster about clothing, cleanliness or doing chores, as well as about being "fresh" or
staying out too late may become conspicuous issues. Withdrawn
or aggressive behavior, as well as arrogance and bossiness, may be
critical problems. Lying, stealing and other antisocial acts, especially when these are carried out recklessly and ostentatiously, suggest a trend toward delinquency and arouse intense forebodings of
disaster for both the family and the youthful offender.

In the past, such problems brought far more boys than girls to
psychiatric attention, but a more even distribution between the
sexes is increasingly apparent.

Other common complaints center on learning difficulties. In view
of the stepped-up requirements confronting the child as he enters
either junior high school or high school, and the disgrace associated
with scholastic failure in these schools, such problems may create
grave concern.

Sources of Referral

The source of the referral may be strongly indicative of the nature
of a child's problem. A referral by school authorities is likely to
signify either learning difficulties or inappropriate behavior in the
restricted confines of a classroom. A referral by a community recreational center suggests difficulties in interpersonal relationships. If
the referral is made by a juvenile court, it is probable that the
child's acting out has entered the category of delinquency. The fact
that a pediatrician has referred the child for a psychiatric consul-

tation may indicate that, in his periodic contacts with the child, he has become concerned about the persistence or increasing intensity of some psychosomatic condition or behavior problems which the parents themselves have overlooked or condoned.

Any information accompanying referrals from such sources merits the utmost consideration. Since it is based on relatively objective and direct observation of the child, it may prove to be an important supplement to the historical data provided by the parents.

When the source of the referral is the parents themselves, the information given to the psychiatrist must be assessed in terms of the parents' attitudes. Parents who seek psychiatric help for children display a variety of motivations; these can be roughly differentiated as reflecting primarily either concern for the child or the annoyance which his symptoms are causing them. Often, too, both types of motives are present and the examiner has to determine which is dominant. A parent who is deeply concerned about the handicapping effect of the child's symptoms and their implications for his future well-being may also express irritation about the difficulties which he himself is experiencing in living with the youngster, but it will become evident that these are secondary considerations; indeed, his attitude will merely prove that he is a human being. Another parent will focus dramatically on the effects of the symptoms on himself and betray, by his unfeeling reference to the child's present distress or possible future unhappiness, that these are minor matters when measured against his own annoyance. Nevertheless, the very fact that he is bringing the child to professional attention justifies the assumption that the parent desires to cooperate in the efforts to ameliorate his offspring's difficulties. Any genuine concern displayed for the child's own welfare, however secondarily it may figure in the referral, ought to be exploited in the hope that it can be utilized to good advantage in the therapeutic task ahead.

Real and Fancied Problems

One cannot too strongly emphasize that a child's having been referred for treatment, from whatever source, does not in itself signify that he has a real problem. All too often, the decision that a child has a behavior problem is based on nothing more substantial than the fact that someone has lodged a complaint about him, and it must be borne in mind that some complaints are more symptomatic of the complainer than the object of his displeasure. Just as the pediatrician makes his independent determination about the adequacy of a child's diet instead of relying on the judgment of the mother who insists that her youngster doesn't "eat a 'thing," the psychiatrist must satisfy himself that a behavior problem actually does exist before trying to determine what may have caused it. In other words, it is always the psychiatrist, not the person reporting the apparent problem, who makes the diagnosis.

To do so requires, first of all, adequate knowledge of norms of behavior based on age and other pertinent factors. As an illustration, however annoying tantrums may be, they do not constitute abnormal conduct if the child is only two years old; but if he is screaming, kicking and flinging himself on the floor at twelve years of age, he is unquestionably manifesting serious aberration. Again, though a mother may believe that her one year old ought to be able to feed himself, most babies of that age are incapable of such self-sufficiency. Similarly, parents who interpret a youngster's normal struggles with some of his school studies as evidence of extraordinary difficulties may have to be made aware of the slow pace at which initial learning sometimes proceeds.

One must also explore the possibility, in dealing with a presumed behavior problem, that the pattern of action may represent an appropriate response to the environment. Hostility and even belligerent conduct may prove to be a justifiable reaction to an unfriendly or highly provoking situation.

SELECTED REFERENCES

Leighton, A. H.: *My Name Is Legion,* New York, Basic Books, 1959.
Lemkau, P. V.: *Mental Hygiene in Public Health.* New York, McGraw-Hill, 1955.
Macmillian, A. M.: *The Health Opinion Survey: Technique for Estimating Prevalence of Psychoneurotic and Related Types of Disorder in Communities. Psychological Reports, Monograph Supplement No. 7.* Birmingham, Ala., Southern Universities Press, 1957.
Pasamanick, B., and Knobloch, H.: Retrospective studies on the epidemiology of reproductive casualty: Old and new. *Merrill-Palmer Quart.* 12:7-23, 1966.
Shaw, C. R.: *The Psychiatric Disorders of Childhood.* New York, Appleton-Century-Crofts, 1966.
Srole, L. et al.: *Mental Health in the Metropolis.* New York, McGraw-Hill, 1962.
Thomas, A., Chess, S., and Birch, H. G.: *Temperament and Behavior Disorders in Children.* New York, New York University Press, 1968.

5. Taking the History

THE HISTORY-TAKING PROCESS is crucial for assessing the behavioral problems of children. In child psychiatry, as in any other branch of medicine, a well-taken history gives clues to diagnosis and indicates what further laboratory and clinical data should be sought. A step-by-step inquiry into a child's development may reveal the origins of his disturbance and make possible an efficient approach to its amelioration.

Yet there has been a persistent tendency to downgrade history-taking in child psychiatry. Many clinicians feel, as Allen (1942) put it, that "a good history is one that grows naturally out of the case," and that a child's problem may be obscured by a "cold set of facts" drawn up in an initial session. Other psychiatrists maintain that the history is inevitably subjective and therefore unreliable as a basis for diagnosis.

In my own experience, the history has proved to be an essential component of the diagnostic evaluation. To be sure, it is only the first stage and cannot be taken as conclusive. The diagnostic process also includes the clinical interview with the child and the use of supplementary fact-finding procedures. These later stages will be discussed in the chapters that follow.

It is true, of course, that behavior is usually reported in subjective terms. But the psychiatrist, as a physician, has been trained to evaluate subjective symptomatology in physical illness, and this training can be put to good use.

When a patient complains of pain, for example, he is making a completely subjective report; no outsider can affirm or deny the presence of painful sensation. Nevertheless, the physician customarily proceeds to delineate the facts motivating such a complaint by ascertaining specific details. He asks questions such as the following: Is it a sharp pain or a dull one? Do you feel it in just one spot, or does it radiate? What relieves it? Are you feeling this pain more frequently than you did in the past? Does it come at regular intervals? By the deliberate formulation of his questions, the physi-

cian is able to convert a subjective complaint into a pattern suggestive of diagnostic possibilities. Behavior problems can be delineated
in the same organized and objective manner.

When parents designate certain types of behavior as problems,
they are imposing their own value judgments. Whether the story
be told in psychologically sophisticated or naive phraseology, the
informant will tend to focus on psychodynamics: the patient's
relationship with the members of his family, feeling tones, issues of
empathy, hostility, resentments, and many other intangibles. By
asking relevant and, if necessary, persistent questions, the psychiatrist must attempt to pin down subjective descriptions to concrete
statements and to shift the emphasis from interpretations to facts.

The following case studies demonstrate the possibility of hearing
two histories in which the parents' interpretations of their roles
appeared similar but were actually very different. Each set of
parents expressed guilt over their early handling of the child. They
felt that they were totally responsible for his present behavior disorder because they had rejected him. Each child was irritable in
infancy, had eating difficulties, was fed forcibly for a period, and
was left periodically in the care of surrogate mothers.

In the first case, further investigation during the parental interview revealed that this child, both in the newborn nursery and
under the care of the baby nurse at home, had been extremely
irritable, had very unclear patterns of sleep and hunger, and had
been sensitive to every noise, touch sensation, or position change.
The parental "rejection," on further inquiry, actually turned out
to be parental feelings of inadequacy. These had arisen as the baby,
their first born, failed to respond to the care given him. He did not
gain weight, and he wailed constantly. This easy irritability was
characteristic throughout his entire eight years. In the child's first
eighteen months, there was a constant shift in mother substitutes:
a succession of nurses, each of whom left after a brief period because
the child was so difficult and unresponsive to their care. A forced-
feeding episode, limited to one week, occurred after the very
thin nine month old infant had lost several pounds and his mother
became panicky about his state of emaciation. It was felt, in this
case, that the parents' self-recriminations were not appropriate.

In the second case, it appeared that the child was unwanted
because he came too soon after a sister, who was suffering from

eczema and needed much care. The infant fared well during his first six months under the regimes of a baby nurse and, later, his grandmother. When the mother assumed the baby's care, she was impatient and, begrudging the time "stolen" from the needs of her older child, dumped him whenever possible on the father. The father had no liking for such an assignment and obtained no pleasure from it. Sleep disturbances and mealtime battles began at that time, setting the pattern for the continuing parent-child hostility. Eventually, neither parent could manage this negativistic child, who was turned over to the care of nurses and baby sitters as often as possible. In this case, the parents' feelings of guilt over their early rejection of the child appeared to be completely justified.

Scope of Historical Data

For the concept that psychiatric problems must be viewed as a continuum of the past and present, we are largely indebted to Sigmund Freud and Adolf Meyer. Both men pointed up the necessity for taking an etiologic approach to a present difficulty, and it was Meyer's concept of psychobiology that led to the introduction of organized history-taking.

What kind of information should be included in the history? Wendell Muncie (1948) recommended that it encompass the present illness, past history, personality and family history. Should the data become too complicated, Meyer (1950) suggested drawing up a life chart on which events are juxtaposed in their proper time sequence and relationship.

At the Institute for Child Guidance in New York City, an important training and treatment center early in the child guidance movement (1927-1933), history-taking was considered to be an essential part of the diagnostic study. David M. Levy (1964), director of the clinic, points out that history-taking followed this general plan: The interview was so structured as to produce a good life history and equivalent data for all records. Time was allowed for spontaneous elaboration by the informant. It was considered necessary to bring up early in the interview the problem for which the child was referred. Hence, any issues about which the mother was particularly concerned were certain to be covered.

Leo Kanner (1957) feels that history-taking is a means of getting to know a person as well as of collecting data. He prefers not to use an outline, but to begin with a type of general question that permits the mother to present the child's problems as she views them and to make her account as subjective and discursive as she wishes. Kanner believes that this makes it possible to gain some understanding of the parental attitudes and conflicts as well as interrelationships within the family. He completes the history with two series of questions—the first on the family history and the second on the personal history of the child. By this process he obtains what he regards as the essential factual data as well as a further exposition of the informant's attitudes.

Anna Freud (1965) employs a "metaphysical" profile of a child which includes data on organic, psychic, environmental, innate and historical elements; traumatic and beneficial events, past and present development, behavior, achievements, successes and failures, defenses and symptomatology. In her judgment, this comprehensive profile can be drawn up at a preliminary diagnostic stage (at the first contact between child and clinic), during analysis (treatment stage), and after (terminal stage).

Various outlines and schemes have been employed by other workers, but a history form is no better than the person using it. Merely amassing facts does not automatically lead to their comprehension. On the other hand, it is possible to gather facts with discrimination and to use them purposefully; there need be no conflict between having a complete form and using it skillfully.

Participation of Parents

To compile a meaningful history of a child, one must turn for information to the adults who play major roles in his life, usually his mother and father. On occasion, the presence of a third informant—perhaps a grandmother—may be warranted; in other special circumstances, the mother and stepfather or the father and a housekeeper will delineate the salient points. In some instances, parents who have been separated or divorced may come to an interview together and apply themselves amicably to the solution of their child's problems.

Although the practice of taking the history from the mother alone is common and often appears to be the most feasible, it is not to be recommended. Whenever possible, the father should also be included in the initial interview. A history taken from the mother alone may seem more unified than one based on information from two or more persons who disagree on certain points, but the latter is the more meaningful history. Two forthright expositions of the contradictory attitudes that influenced the child are more illuminating than the presentation of one parent's view. This is especially true when the absent parent is blamed for all the negative factors in the child's environment. If a single parent is the informant, one is likely to get not only a biased account of the child's behavior, but also a distorted evaluation of the child's relationship with the other parent.

We are interested, moreover, in the parents' relationship with each other and how it has influenced their handling of the child. When both parents participate, any antagonism they feel toward each other usually becomes obvious before the interview is concluded, even if they were on their company behavior when they arrived. The nature of their relationship is revealed in countless ways—in how they try to verify the accuracy of their recollections, in how they air differences of opinion and react to each other's criticisms as well as in all the by-play incidental to remembering data and describing the child's patterns of response. The joint interview may reveal the dominance of one parent and the submissiveness of the other, contemptuous attitudes and exploitativeness. Generally, more can be learned about the shortcomings and strengths of the parents by posing questions about factual details than by focusing directly on attitudes.

One should guard against making facile judgments about the parents' personalities from an impression gathered when they are under stressful circumstances. In investigating the troublesome behavior of the child, one may tap mainly negative aspects of expressed attitudes and relationships. Sometimes the parents themselves become aware of this and interrupt themselves to say, "We are only telling the negative side; our daughter is also charming and intelligent when she isn't having a tantrum." If the history-taker fails to ask about nonproblem aspects of behavior, he may get a one-sided picture that omits the parent's positive interactions with the child.

Nor should the interviewer assume that attitudes currently expressed by the parents have always been present. Sometimes a parent spontaneously reports shifts in attitude. For example, in discussing a child who stole money, balked at routines and lied habitually, one mother said that the behavior pattern had improved, largely because her approach to the child had undergone a marked change during the past year. She had previously resented the child as ugly and cantankerous, identifying her strongly with the divorced father. At the urging of her second husband, the mother attempted to change her attitude. At first she did this mechanically. But when the child responded positively to the new approach, the mother began to find pleasure in her daughter's company and described her as having become pretty, intelligent and often helpful. The mother requested the consultation to find out if she was doing everything possible to maintain this positive trend, and to help her root out any lingering negative attitudes and destructive handling.

This spontaneous reporting of a changed parental attitude is understandable when a positive trend develops in the child-parent interaction. Under other circumstances, however, parents may not be as keenly aware of their attitudes or of alterations in them. Indeed, in a deteriorating interaction, with a negative parental stance arising in part from the child's behavior difficulties, one may easily overlook the existence of earlier positive attitudes. It is the history-taker's responsibility to search for them.

The parents' personalities may be clearly revealed only in the way they respond to specific recommendations for child handling. Unexpected flexibilities or rigidities may give insight into the parents' role in the parent-child interchange.

A parent's inability to recall significant developmental dates, or his ignorance about norms of development, may reveal a casual, indifferent or rejecting attitude toward the child. A marked tendency to interpret information instead of presenting it factually may reveal personal bias. The manner in which a serious illness is recalled will give useful clues to a parent's ability to mobilize himself effectively to meet an emergency as well as to withdraw, once it is over, the special measures of protection that are no longer warranted.

The accuracy of parental recall may be crucial in determining one's ability to understand and diagnose the child's behavior problem. Past events are often recollected in the service of current comprehensions, hopes and fears. Such factual data as the ages at which the child began to walk and talk, or was toilet-trained, tend to be inaccurately remembered when they have deviated from what the parents consider the average or desirable age. The onset of certain behavior patterns will often be misdated to conform with presuppositions derived from popular views in psychiatry. For example, one pair of parents claimed that a child's problem dated back to the birth of a younger brother, thus proving that "sibling rivalry" was the culprit. But in this case anterospective data were available to check the memory, and the problem had actually been present a full year before the sibling was born. While it is not always possible to spot such inaccuracies, the parent's statements should be cross-checked for inconsistencies.

When parents are interviewed separately, their statements on some matters may be so contradictory as to preclude any reliance on the history as recorded by each. Moreover, the report of an interview with the psychiatrist given by one parent to the other may so distort or even contradict the essence of what the psychiatrist meant to convey that the possibility of helping the child may be lost. Even when there is no deliberate attempt to misrepresent, the substance of what comes out of the interview is too often interpreted solely in the light of the hopes, needs and desires of the parent who is present. This is especially apt to happen if the diagnosis or advice given is unpalatable. In fact, if roadblocks are erected to prevent the history-taker from meeting the absent parent, one may assume that the parents sharply disagree about their child's behavior disorder, and that the recommendations will be distorted or the consultation itself converted into ammunition for a parental battle.

Later, however, it may become advisable to confer privately with one parent, especially if that parent—with or without the knowledge of the other—requests such a consultation. A private interview may lead to disclosures concerning the personality difficulties of one spouse, or the request for an interview may have been made for the purpose of discussing mental illness in the family history of either of them. A parent who desires to disclose such facts privately may be motivated by genuine respect and consideration for the marital partner, or he may find it easier to discuss these facts by himself. Strong feelings of resentment or even of hostility brewing in one parent may be difficult to express in the other's presence; or descriptions of a spouse's extremely destructive attitudes may be withheld in fear of painful retaliatory measures. For these and many other reasons, a parent's attempt to arrange for a private discussion should not be discouraged, and the occasion should then be utilized to obtain a fuller and more accurate assessment of the relevant factors.

Using the History Guide

The history form reproduced on pages 70-72 is presented as a guide to the history-taking and a reminder of the factual areas that are important to explore. Of course, the form is to be used selectively, since it would never be completed if the history-taker attempted to go through each area of investigation with a fine-tooth comb. In any specific case, some aspects of the history may be vitally important and others relatively insignificant, depending upon the nature of the problems presented by an individual patient. As in exploring a physical condition, an awareness of the diagnostic possibilities will signal the areas in which detailed data should be obtained.

If a child has an educational problem, for example, it may be essential to get full school and developmental histories, while the data on health will yield little information pertinent to his difficulties. On the other hand, a youngster with a syndrome of strong hostility and dependency may have been influenced to an extraordinary degree by an early illness that required heroic nursing care over a long period. The parents' ages when the child was born, or the amount of time that elapsed between their marriage and the birth of the child, may be either inconsequential or highly significant for understanding the case. It must also be borne in mind that entries on normal development or superior functioning in certain areas may be as vital for delineating a problem as notations about inadequate functioning in other areas. Moreover, since a history focusing on specific difficulties may tend to give a distorted impression of the youngster's personality, one should make a special effort to obtain a description of the child as a total personality. This would include gathering specific information on his temperamental characteristics. The value of each completed form as a diagnostic tool is determined in large measure by the skill and foresightedness of the history-taker. The form calls for information about the young patient in a number of general categories. These are discussed below.

Referral

As noted earlier, the identity of the person (or persons) serving as the link between the psychiatrist and those who are consulting him about the child may be of more than *pro forma* significance for the case. A referral through a friend of the family usually indicates that the parents are concerned about the child's problems. When a school, a social agency or a playground director refers the case, a specific area of maladjustment is probably involved. Sometimes the referral is by a pediatrician. Since he suggested the consultation, he may be a source of valuable information on the behavior and upbringing of the child and on the intrafamily relationships, as well as on any general health problems.

Identifying Data

The biographic information helps to orient the psychiatrist to the child, his immediate family and his social milieu. Even seemingly insignificant details may be important here. For example, the given names of the patient and his sibs may convey something about the family. Some parents tend to address a child by a nickname. Others give their offspring rather cumbersome names, which they enunciate most precisely, thereby indicating a certain formality or distance in the family structure.

Information on the parents' occupations (including the mother's previous occupation if she has become a full-time homemaker) gives some notion of the cultural standards maintained in their home and of the educational and social concepts that the young patient has been absorbing since his early days. The youngster whose family functions on a high cultural level should not be regarded as a genius every time a four-syllable word rolls off his tongue, whereas a child from a culturally impoverished home who possesses a rich vocabulary gives evidence of being extremely alert. On the other hand, if the vocabulary of one brought up in the latter type of home is extremely limited, that fact might be accepted merely as a reflection of his surroundings rather than as a reliable indicator of the child's intellectual capacity.

Data on the patient's sibs will help to clarify his own position in the family hierarchy and will alert the history-taker to the existence of any special stresses or strains produced by that position. Unusual facts about each sib, and about any other children who may be permanent members of the household, should also be secured.

Presenting Problems

The tone of the entire relationship between the parents and the psychiatrist is usually set by how the psychiatrist obtains information on the presenting problems. Parents arriving at the psychiatrist's office usually have some preconceived notions about their role in the situation and appear generally discomforted by it. They may be worried, defensive, guilt-ridden, angry, annoyed, or, less often, appropriately concerned and open-minded. Their initial report of the child's symptoms and behavior will usually suggest further points to be looked into and other questions to be put. As these problems are presented one after another, they may appear to constitute different facets of the same basic difficulty; a fairly consistent behavior pattern often emerges from the discussion.

For example, the parents may report a series of complaints: a teacher says that the child annoys his classmates; the neighbors comment that he is constantly picking fights with their children; and parents themselves assert that the child cannot be kept from fighting with his sibs. The child may also be described as unreliable: he does whatever comes into his head without any regard for the consequences; he is accident-prone; he destroys household objects or his own possessions. All of these particulars create a graphic portrait of a hyperactive, impulsive child whose clash with his environment takes varied forms under different circumstances, though all are rooted in the same underlying problem.

One informant relating this entire series of difficulties will tend to make light of the effect of the child's behavior on others and may criticize teachers or neighbors who have made an issue of it. Criticism of this nature is apt to be especially sharp when the family has been subjected to strong pressure to bring the child under psychiatric care. Yet this informant may also be unable to conceal his own annoyance over the child's conduct at home. Another parent bringing up similar problems may manifest deep concern over the effect of his child's behavior on others, and appear to take personal responsibility for any trouble he is causing. A third parent may focus on his own interpretation of his child's pathologic conduct, exhibiting either smug satisfaction that he was able to trace it back to its origin or much guilt because he regards himself as the major cause of the difficulty.

The marked differences in parental attitudes indicate the advisability of pinning down an informant's general statement about a problem with concrete illustrations, even requesting a "blow by blow" account of a characteristic episode. Generalities often prove to have been more descriptive of a parent's frame of mind than of a child's behavior. The flat statement that a little girl has no confidence in herself may refer equally well to one who is shy or retiring, to one who gives up easily rather than face an anticipated failure, to a boastful and bossy youngster, or to a child who cannot tolerate criticism.

As the pattern of the child's interaction with the environment becomes clearer, the history-taker can make a mental note to pursue certain lines of inquiry. In the case of the hyperactive, impulsive child, for example, a scrutiny of the obstetric and medical history would be in order, to investigate the possibility that this is a child with cerebral dysfunction. The child's temperamental attributes in infancy also need to be looked into.

From the order in which complaints are given and the relative emphasis which the father and mother place on each complaint, it is possible to obtain not only a picture of the child but also a preliminary impression of the parental attitudes. If the parents focus on the difficulties that the child's behavior is creating for them, the approach to therapy promises to be less constructive than if they emphasize the effects of the child's disturbance on his own development and well-being. It should be remembered, however, that parents genuinely concerned about their child are justified, too, in having some consideration for themselves; their recognition of the annoying nature of certain symptoms should not in itself be construed as rejection of the child.

From the parents' initial listing of problems and their explanation of why they are seeking help, the psychiatrist may also obtain
valuable insight into their readiness to accept real responsibilities
for an appropriate resolution of the behavioral difficulty. A tendency to heap coals of fire on one's own head rarely leads to the
constructive reexamination of past events and relationships on
which any new approach to a problem must be based. Immersing
oneself in guilt more often leads to the avoidance of responsibility
than to its assumption, since one may well expend all one's energy
in discharging the intense guilt feelings. The opposite attitude—
that of blaming the neighbors, playmates and teachers for the child's
problems—is certainly no better approach to an examination of a
parent's own role in creating or maintaining a destructive situation.

In the investigation of each problem presented, it is important to
ascertain its duration, the circumstances which seem to have
initiated or contributed to its development, whether or not it is
recurrent, and the relative intensity of the present manifestations.

Birth and Infancy

Having recorded the presenting problems, the history-taker is
ready to probe into the past for what light it can shed on them.
The parents' ages and the length of the marriage at the time of the
child's birth may contribute to an understanding of the atmosphere
into which he was born. It is important to note facts such as that
a child was born out of wedlock or after the parents had been
childless for many years. A striking discrepancy in the ages of the
parents or the information that both were no longer youthful
when the child was born may highlight the existence of special
anxieties or incompatibility in motives and ideas, any of which
may prove to be crucial data for further investigation.

The number of times the mother was pregnant before the patient
was conceived, and the ratio of her healthy children to miscarriages, stillbirths or living children with congenital anomalies may
point up possibilities of subclinical, organic factors in the child
as well as explain special family attitudes, such as intense fears or
expectations centered in the child. If a defect in another sib or
in the young patient himself is of known familial origin, its possible
effects should be explored with the parents.

But one must not assume an automatic correlation between certain factual data and attitudinal implications. A long hiatus between the date of the marriage and the birth of the first child could be due to factors such as low fertility; a series of miscarriages with the possibility of deviant fetal development; negative parental attitudes toward having children; or financial difficulties during the early years of the marriage. In any of these eventualities, the data may provide a vital clue to behavioral difficulties or may add little or nothing to an understanding of the family picture.

The history of the mother's pregnancy, labor and delivery, as well as data on the child's weight at birth and events of the neonatal period, may reveal the presence of early organic difficulties. Entries about the infant's care should note who took care of him. Details of the feeding history should include whether he was breast-fed or bottle-fed, the age at which weaning began and the time required for its completion, and comment on the introduction of new foods and the development of self-feeding.

Whether a baby was breast-fed or bottle-fed may or may not be significant. Bottle-feeding represents an aspect of the urban middle-class pattern of infant care today. Many authorities on child care have in the past tended to equate bottle-feeding with maternal rejection. Although such a conclusion may have been more or less warranted at a time when bottle-feeding was an exceptional procedure, in the social group in which it represents the norm such a practice bears little or no relation to maternal attitudes. A mother who at the present time has a strong desire to breast-feed her baby actually may find herself going counter to the regular routine of her obstetrician and the newborn nursery. Even information about how much the child was held during the course of his bottle-feeding may shed more light on the number of children his mother had to care for and her equal concern for all of them than on the quality of her relatedness to this particular child during his infancy. It may be anticipated that fewer bottles were propped up for the firstborn than for those who followed. The child's individual style of indicating hunger, satiation and food preferences, and the mother's response to his behavior are all aspects of the feeding history that may be instructive. The interview should also note the child's reaction to restrictive or unpalatable diets that may have been medically prescribed.

Recommended techniques and schedules for weaning a baby vary from one generation to the next. Even within the same generation, pediatricians, psychiatrists and other child-care specialists may have very different notions of the "optimum moment." The various theories have in common little more than the certainty with which each is advocated as it becomes fashionable. One generation of specialists may regard it as very undesirable for an infant to be on the bottle after he is ten months old, whereas the next generation may warn that weaning him to the cup before he is eighteen months old will have a disastrous effect on the developing personality.

It is important to learn which person or combination of persons was responsible for the baby's day-to-day care. If the mother was employed outside the home or had another outside responsibility, one should investigate how this affected her relationship with the baby and his daily schedule. One cliché judgment voiced repeatedly equates the working mother with the rejecting mother, but there is no reliable evidence to substantiate this hypothesis.

The next series of entries on the form comprise a developmental study. This encompasses vital steps in maturation, i.e., the ages at which the child became capable of sitting, standing, walking, saying his first word, and also the salient facts about his toilet training. The information in this category often gives valuable clues to diagnosis.

A significant lag in motor maturation may point either to specific neurologic difficulties, which may not have been previously recognized, or to mental retardation. The combination of such a lag with normal or precocious development in language would suggest that the cause is something other than mental retardation. On the other hand, extreme variability in the pattern of language development and a delay in speech itself do not necessarily imply that the general intellectual development was sluggish.

Even children of normal or superior intelligence may not utter their first word until they are two and a half years old; characteristically, in that case, a speedy pick-up in language function follows so that, within a short period of time, it is impossible to distinguish such children from those who started to speak earlier. Where a whole speech pattern is uniformly delayed—no babbling during infancy, no exploration of sounds during the first eighteen months, the first word spoken after the age of three, and thereafter a very gradual development in the use of language—one would suspect that the delay has been caused either by general retardation or a specific maturational lag in the area of language.

Temperament in Infancy

Following the taking of a basic clinical history, systematic inquiry can be made into the child's temperamental characteristics during infancy. The inquiry can be started with a broad question: "After you brought the baby home from the hospital and in the first few weeks and months of his life, what was he like?"

First answers to such questions are usually very general: "He was wonderful," "He cried day and night," "He was a bundle of nerves."

The next question is still open ended: "Would you give me some details that will describe what you mean?"

Replies to this question often include useful descriptions of behaviors from which judgments of temperament may be made. Further information requires specific inquiry, which is most economically pursued by taking up areas of behavior relevant to each of the temperamental attibutes one at a time. The questions should be directed at obtaining descriptive behavioral items from which the interviewer can make an estimate of the child's temperamental characteristics. Here is a list of suggested questions appropriate to each of the temperamental categories.

Activity Level.—How much did your baby move around? Did he move around a lot, was he very quiet, or moderately so? If you put him to bed for a nap and it took him ten or fifteen minutes to fall asleep, would you have to go in to rearrange the covers, or would he be lying so quietly that you knew they would not be disarranged? If you were changing his diaper and discovered that you had left the powder just out of reach, could you safely dash over to get it and come right back without worrying that he would flip over the surface and fall? Did you have trouble changing his diaper, pulling his shirt over his head or putting on any other of his clothing because he wiggled about, or could you count on his lying quietly to be dressed?

Rhythmicity.—How did you arrange the baby's feedings? Could you tell by the time he was six weeks (two months, three months) old about when during the day he would be hungry, sleepy or wake up? Could you count on this happening about the same time every day or did the baby vary from day to day? If there was variation, how marked was it? About when during the day did he have his bowel movements (time and number) and was this routine variable or predictable?

Parents can generally recall such events. They will say, "He was regular as clockwork," "I could never figure out when to start a long job because one day he would have a long nap and the next day he wouldn't sleep more than fifteen minutes," or, "I used to try to take him out for his airing after I cleaned him from his bowel movement, but I never could figure it right because his time changed every day."

Adaptability.—How did the child respond to changed circumstances? When he was shifted from a bathinette to a bathtub, did he take to the change immediately? If not, could you count on his getting used to it quickly or did it take a long time? (Parents should be asked to define what they mean by "quickly" and what they mean by "a long time" in terms of days or weeks.) If his first reaction to a new person was a negative one, how long did it take the child to become familiar with the person? If he didn't like a new food the first time it was offered, could you count on his getting to like it and most other new foods sooner or later? If so, how long would it take if the new food was offered to him daily or several times a week?

Approach—Withdrawal.—How did the baby behave with new events, such as when he was given his first tub bath, offered new foods or taken care of by an unfamiliar person? Did he fuss, did he do nothing, or did he seem to like it? Were there any changes during his infancy that you remember, such as a shift to a new bed, or a visit to a new place? Describe the child's initial behavior at these times.

Threshold Level.—How would you estimate the baby's sensitivity to noises, heat and cold, things he saw and tasted, and textures of clothing? Did he seem very aware of these things or unresponsive? Did you have to tiptoe about when the baby was sleeping lest he be awakened? If he heard a faint noise while awake, would he tend to notice the sound by looking toward it? Did bright lights or bright sunshine make him blink or cry? Did the baby's behavior seem to show that he noticed the difference when a familiar person wore glasses or a new hair style for the first time in his presence? If he didn't like a new food and if an old food that he liked very much was put with it on the spoon, would the baby still notice the taste of the new one and reject it?

Intensity of Reaction.—How did you know when the baby was hungry? Did he squeak, did he roar, or were his sounds somewhere in between? How could you tell that he didn't like a food? Did he just quietly turn his head away from the spoon or did he start crying loudly? If you held his hand to cut his fingernails and he didn't like it, did he fuss a little or a lot? If he liked something, did he usually smile and coo or did he laugh loudly? In general, would you say he let his pleasure or displeasure be known loudly or softly?

Quality of Mood.—How could you tell when the baby liked something or disliked something? (After a description of the infant's behavior in these respects is obtained, the parents should be asked if he was more often contented or more often discontented and on what basis they made this judgment.)

Distractibility.—If the child was sucking on the bottle or breast, would he stop when he heard a sound or if another person came by, or would he continue sucking? If he was hungry and fussing or crying while the bottle was being warmed, could you divert him easily and stop his crying by holding him or giving him a plaything? If he was playing—for example, gazing at his fingers or using a rattle—would other sights and sounds get his attention very quickly or very slowly?

Persistence and Attention Span.—Would you say that the baby usually stuck with something he was doing for a long time or only momentarily? For example, describe the longest time he remained engrossed in an activity all by himself. How old was he and what was he doing? (Examples might be playing with the cradle gym or watching a mobile.) If he reached for something, say a toy in the bathtub, and couldn't get it easily, would he keep after it or give up very quickly?

Temperament at Later Stages of Development

After completing the inventory of the child's temperamental characteristics in infancy, the next step is to identify those attributes which appear extreme in their manifestations and those which seem clearly related to the child's current pattern of deviant behavior. This is followed by an inquiry into the expression of these temperamental attributes at succeeding age-stage periods of development. Thus, if the history of the infancy period suggests a pattern of marked distractibility, it is desirable to gather data on behavior related to distractibility at succeeding age periods and in varied life situations, such as play, school or homework. Similarly, if the presenting complaints indicate that the child currently finds it difficult to undertake new activities or to join new groups of age-mates, and if the early temperamental history suggests a characteristic pattern of initial withdrawal coupled with slow adaptation, it is important to obtain descriptions of his initial responses to situations and demands at various points in his developmental course.

The final step in assessing the child's temperament is the evaluation of his current temperamental characteristics. The information obtained for current functioning is usually more valid than that obtained for past patterns of behavior, since the problems of forgetting and retrospective distortion are minimized. The inquiry into present behavior, while attempting to cover all temperamental categories, should concentrate on those which appear most pertinent to the presenting symptoms.

Activity level may be estimated from a child's behavior preferences. Would he rather sit quietly for a long time engrossed in some task or does he prefer to seek out opportunities for active physical play? How does he fare in routines that require sitting still for extended periods of time? For example, can he sit through an entire meal without seeking an opportunity to move about? Must a long train or automobile ride be broken up by frequent stops because of his restlessness?

Adaptability can be identified through a consideration of the way the child reacts to changes in environment. Does he adjust easily and fit quickly into changed family patterns? Does he have difficulty adapting to the routines of a new classroom or a new teacher? Is he willing to go along with other children's preferences or does he always insist on pursuing only his own interests?

Approach-withdrawal, or the youngster's pattern of response to new events and people, can be explored in many ways. Questions can be directed at the nature of his reaction to new clothing, new neighborhood children, a new school, and a new teacher. What is his attitude when a family excursion is being planned? Will he readily try new foods or activities?

Threshold level is more difficult to explore in an older child than in a young one. However, it is sometimes possible to obtain information on unusual features of threshold, such as hypersensitivity to noise, visual stimuli and rough clothing, or remarkable unresponsiveness to such stimuli.

The intensity of reactions can be ascertained by finding out how the child displays disappointment or pleasure. If something pleasant happens, does he tend to be mildly enthusiastic, average in his expression of joy, or ecstatic? When he is unhappy, does he fuss quietly or bellow with rage or distress?

Quality of mood can usually be estimated by parental descriptions of their offspring's over-all expressions of mood. Is he predominantly happy and contented or is he a frequent complainer and more often unhappy than not?

Distractibility, even when not a presenting problem, will declare itself in the parents' descriptions of ordinary routines. Does the child start off to do something and then often get sidetracked by something his brother is doing, by his coin collection or by any number of circumstances that catch his eye or his ear? Or once he is engaged in an activity, is he impervious to what is going on around him?

Data on persistence and attention span are usually easier to obtain for the older child than for the infant. The degree of persistence in the face of difficulty can be ascertained with regard to games, puzzles, athletic activities and school work. Similarly, after the initial difficulty in mastering these activities has been overcome, the length of the child's attention span for and concentration on these same kinds of activities can be ascertained.

The delineation of the child's temperamental characteristics at different age-periods may indicate that changes have occurred over time. There are normal variations of temperament and the fate of any temperamental attribute is dependent upon a host of influences.

The process of socialization may blur the individual behavioral style evident in new situations and experiences. In other words, certain patternings of response, once they are adapted to a cultural norm, may serve to minimize individual variations. For example, the first attempt at toilet-training will cause one child to scream and struggle violently, another to fuss mildly while he sits on the seat for only a few minutes, and a third child to smile and play while sitting on the seat for many minutes. A year later, when all three children are fully trained, their behavior on the toilet seat may show comparatively slight differences.

Similar blurring of initial differences may occur with a variety of other experiences, such as entry into nursery school, the beginning of formal learning, changes in the family group, new living quarters. Therefore, when the behavioral history suggests an apparent change in a child's temperament over time, the data should be scrutinized to determine whether the change remains in evidence or disappears when the responses to new situations at the different age-periods are compared.

In many instances, additional data on temperamental organization can be obtained by querying teachers or other adults familiar with the child's behavior. For such inquiry, the history-taking protocol for the parents can be utilized if it is appropriately modified to permit a focus on the areas of the child's functioning with which the adult is acquainted.

Health

Sufficient headway in outlining diagnostic possibilities has now been made for the history-taker to assess the relevance of data about the child's physical health. To begin with, one would inquire routinely about operations and childhood illnesses and delineate a year-by-year pattern of health or illness. If the data already obtained suggest that the child may have suffered from a borderline cerebral palsy, for example, this possibility should be thoroughly investigated. In such a situation, it may even be in order to go over, once more, the details of the child's motor development to get a precise description of how he sat, crawled or held his body when taking his first steps.

Descriptions of physical illnesses and of how they were dealt with may clearly reveal attitudes of underprotection or overprotection, or may testify to the parents' sensible handling of their child. It may become evident that a child with a slight tendency to asthma is not permitted to play with other youngsters because his mother fears that he may perspire too much. In contrast, the parents of a child with cerebral palsy or other serious illness with permanent sequelae may always have encouraged him to become self-assertive within the limits imposed by the residual handicap. Other parents may have been unable to recognize the serious consequences of illness, expressing annoyance at a child for knocking things over even though this was the result of disturbed motor coordination.

Wherever possible, the psychiatrist should obtain confirming reports of physical illnesses recalled by the informants. Medical data supplied by parents may not be completely trustworthy for a number of reasons. Lacking medical knowledge, parents may recollect symptoms which, though important to them, were relatively insignificant in terms of the disease process. The child's physician may have shielded the parents from a full diagnosis of a critical illness or one with morbid sequelae. Some parents deliberately withhold medical data out of shame or fear.

It is also possible that a pediatrician may have put out of his mind certain implications noted in an otherwise minor illness that are recalled only under questioning by the psychiatrist. A case of measles followed by a period of lethargy or high fever may have been carefully watched by a physician who was concerned about the possibility of a complicating encephalitis, and this may never have been mentioned to the parents. If the child's presenting problems appear to resemble a postencephalitic behavior disorder, a direct inquiry made to the pediatrician may provide information of which the parents are totally unaware.

Reports on any previously conducted psychiatric examinations or psychologic tests should also be obtained whenever possible. Parents who have "shopped around" among psychiatrists may be reluctant to have the present consultant examine previous findings, fearing that he will be influenced by a "bad" opinion. Nevertheless, it is important to get information about earlier examinations of the child, just as one would wish to compare a newly taken electrocardiogram with previous ones in order to assess the exact significance of the latest reading. The opinions of earlier psychiatric investigators do not have to be accepted uncritically, but a careful study of their findings will usually tell a great deal about the course of the child's behavior. Indeed, a longitudinal study of a child may

be approximated through such reports, even though the present
consultant has just begun to handle the case.

School History

The information obtained about the child's schooling usually
conveys an impression of his adjustment to other children and to
the learning process. A child presumed to have been normal in
every respect may give the first indication of behavior problems
when he enters an organized group. The parents may have become
so used to adapting themselves to him that they failed to realize
that he would experience some difficulty in adjusting to social
situations, to sharing objects or attention with other children, and
to fighting for his rights. A child whose personal reactions seemed
alert to his parents may be revealed as mentally retarded when he
begins to function for the first time in a formal learning situation.
Data of this sort can contribute significantly to an understanding
of the presenting problems.

Remaining Entries

The remaining items on the history form need only brief discussion. They give the psychiatrist an opportunity to build upon
information already secured or to raise pertinent points requiring
further emphasis. One should already have obtained a good idea
of the patient's relationships with other members of his family and
with his playmates, but it often proves useful to explore what his
parents have to say about these relationships. In probing for additional factors, one should ask the parents if anything of importance
has been overlooked.

At this point in the interview, the examiner may have become
aware of patterns that were not evident earlier. More precise inquiry into the nature of the behavior disorder may now become
possible. The final entry on "impression of parents" might include
observations on the parents' ambitions for the child. It would be
pertinent to record facts such as that one mother showed special
anxiety about her child's penny stealing because one of his uncles
served a jail sentence for embezzlement, and another mother was
afraid to have any more children because her child's problems might
be hereditary.

In assessing all the information obtained on parental attitudes, the history-taker should bear in mind that attitudes change with time. As noted earlier in this chapter, the present attitudes of parents and others taking part in the care of a child should be clearly distinguished from the possibly very different attitudes— even of the same persons—that influenced the child during the earliest years of his life.

In addition, one should be aware of the special circumstances that may influence the formation of parental attitudes. A mother who serenely planned to begin her family when her marital situation was stable may give birth to a child at a moment when her husband is being shipped overseas for military duty or when she has to face serious illness. Such problems may result in her being a far less patient mother than she would have been if her infant had been born, say, a year earlier or several years later. On the other hand, a pregnancy that was most unwelcome may lead to a complete about-face in attitude after a delightful infant has transformed a gloomy household into a joyful one.

It must also be remembered that adverse parental attitudes may have been formed because a child is exceedingly difficult to manage. The attitudes may be the effect rather than the cause of the behavior problems. As Anna Freud (1965) has observed, the psychiatrist "has to exercise great care so as not to be misled by surface appearances and, above all, not to confuse the effect of a child's abnormality on the mother with the mother's pathogenic influence on the child."

Arrangements for the Diagnostic Study

The comprehensive investigation into the patient's history ranges from routine and easy-to-obtain data to subtle influences upon the child's character structure that are far more difficult to explore. By using the history form flexibly and resourcefully, it should be possible to record the history in less than an hour, usually from 45 to 50 minutes. If more time is required, it is well to continue the session until the history has been recorded in full.

Where is the subject of this discussion while the facets of his life are being communicated? Anywhere else but in my waiting

room, if I have my way. Making a child sit behind closed doors
while he is under discussion can intensify whatever problems are
being revealed in the other room. Unless there is some compelling
reason to make special arrangements for the child to be examined
immediately after the history has been taken, his diagnostic study
takes place at a later date, perhaps at the second visit in a three-visit
diagnostic workup. The interval between the visits is not fixed; the
second is arranged at the mutual convenience of the psychiatrist and
the informants. However, the third visit, for further discussion with
the parents and for the making of recommendations, does not take
place until all the medical and psychiatric data and test findings
that are available from other professional sources have been collected and studied. If, for any reason, the psychiatrist feels that
more than one diagnostic interview with the child is needed, this,
too, is scheduled between the taking of this history and the final
session of the diagnostic workup.

When the first stage of this general diagnostic study—the taking
of the history—has been completed, the clinician should have a good
idea of how the child's difficulties ought to be classified. The process
of history taking should provide fruitful clues for first-hand investigation of the child.

HISTORY GUIDE

		Date:	
		Referral:	
Name:	Sex:	Date of Birth:	
Address:			
Father's Name:		Mother's Name:	
Occupation:		Occupation:	
Sibs:	Sex:	Age:	Grade:

Informants:

Presenting Problems:

BIRTH and INFANCY:

Parents' ages when child was born:

Length of marriage when child was born:

Planned baby?   Problems of Conception?

History of pregnancy, labor, and delivery:

Birth weight and neonatal history:

Feeding history:

Daily care of the baby given by:

DEVELOPMENTAL MILESTONES
(AGES OF):

Sitting: Standing: Walking:

1st Word: 1st Phrase or Sentence:

Toilet Training: Time of initiation, mode of procedure:

TEMPERAMENT IN INFANCY:

TEMPERAMENT AT LATER STAGES:

HEALTH:

Operations:

Childhood Diseases:

Other Illnesses:

Accidents:

SCHOOL HISTORY:

Nursery:

Kindergarten:

  1st Grade:

  Present:

INTERPERSONAL RELATIONSHIPS:

ADDITIONAL FACTORS OF IMPORTANCE:

FURTHER DEVELOPMENT OF BEHAVIOR PROBLEMS:

IMPRESSION OF PARENTS:

SELECTED REFERENCES

Allen, F. H.: *Psychotherapy with Children*. New York, W. W. Norton, 1942.
Freud, A.: *Normality and Pathology in Childhood*. New York, International
    Universities Press, 1965.
Kanner, L.: *Child Psychiatry*. Springfield, Ill., Charles C Thomas, 1957.
Levy, D. M.: Modifications of the psychiatric interview. *Amer. J. Psychother.*
    18:435-451, 1964.
Meyer, A.: *Collected Papers of Adolf Meyer*, Winters, E. E. (Ed.). Baltimore, Johns
    Hopkins Press, 1948-1952.
Muncie, W.: *Psychobiology and Psychiatry*. St. Louis, C. V. Mosby, 1948.
Thomas, A., Birch, H. G., Chess, S., Hertzig, M. E., and Korn, S.: *Behavioral
    Individuality in Early Childhood*. New York, New York University Press, 1963.

6. The Diagnostic Interview

AFTER THE HISTORY-TAKING, the second phase of the diagnostic process is the direct interview with the child. There is a wide divergence of opinion about the value of this diagnostic session. Some psychiatrists even doubt that it is necessary.

According to one school of thought, the interview is superfluous because the diagnosis itself, however reached, has no significance for the treatment process; it is "the whole child, not the diagnosis" that is treated. Exponents of this view contend that the therapeutic procedure is the same regardless of the child's specific problem. On the other hand, if one believes that the treatment should be tailored to the behavioral difficulty, the diagnostic interview assumes great importance.

Other psychiatrists, while recognizing the importance of diagnosis, maintain that the interview is unnecessary if an adequate history has been taken. It is true that a comprehensive and accurate psychiatric history will, as a rule, contain useful clues to the child's problems. But even if the interview does no more than confirm and deepen the significance of what has already been learned about the child, it is a vital, indeed indispensable, aspect of the diagnostic process.

For one thing, some of the information reported by parents in the course of history-taking may be colored by their own hopes and fears. The parents' immediate experiences can so affect the focus of their report that it may give the trained observer a quite different impression of the child from the one he obtains in his first direct encounter. An adolescent involved in bitter conflict with his parents, especially if it has been marked by ever-mounting hostility, may exhibit a more reasonable and responsive attitude than could have been predicted from their report of the battle.

The parents' competence to assess the seriousness of behavioral problems is also subject to scrutiny. Some of the difficulties that would appear from the history to justify only mild concern may prove on direct contact with the child to represent highly aberrant conduct and thought processes. The reverse may also be true; a child's personality may be much better integrated than could have been anticipated from the bizarre behavior described in the history. The child who is reported by his parents to be "a little bit slow" may be severely retarded, or he may be manifesting a psychologic defense mechanism, such as an inability to make decisions, which is preventing him from functioning at his full capacity.

Consequently, until the child himself has been seen and evaluated, the diagnosis must be regarded as tentative. In formulating the diagnosis and plan of treatment, the recorded history and the diagnostic interview should be examined together, along with any auxiliary tests or other relevant data.

One purpose of the interview is to decide what further special diagnostic procedures, if any, are required. While completeness is always comforting, costly additional measures should not be demanded lightly. But when they are clearly indicated, the diagnostician should not hesitate to say so. (Supplementary diagnostic procedures are discussed in the next chapter.)

Preliminary Arrangements

The interview with the child should be scheduled for a later date than the one set for the history-taking. A concluding diagnostic consultation with the parents takes place at a third visit, during which observations and recommendations are discussed.

The stage is set for the diagnostic interview at the moment when the child is informed that an appointment has been made for him. While some parents are able to prepare the child appropriately, others may broach the subject in an awkward or even disastrous manner. Hence, advice to parents on how to ready their child for the visit ought to be offered as a regular preliminary routine.

To begin with, the child's age, the severity of the problem, and the quality of his emotional bonds with his parents will determine how he should be informed of the impending visit. It is usually possible to "key" the notification to one or more presenting problems which the child himself would like to overcome, or at least are very much on his mind. The parents may preface their announcement of the appointment by explaining to the child that, in their concern over his difficulty, they have sought a psychiatrist's advice on how they can best help the youngster deal with it. They may go on to say that the psychiatrist, in turn, expressed interest in getting to know him, since it is difficult to give really helpful advice about a person one has never met. Such an explanation will prove to be most constructive when the child has a strong desire to resolve his problem; if, on the other hand, there is hostility toward the parents, such an explanation will be less effective, and an especially tactful approach will be necessary. Obviously, a logical verbal explanation will be meaningless to the very young child. All a three year old requires is the announcement that he will soon be taken on a visit to a playroom where he will find many interesting toys. The child of six or seven may obtain some vague understanding of the approaching interview, though he usually forgets all about the explanation once he is in the playroom engaging in some appropriate activity with the psychiatrist. For the preadolescent or adolescent youngster, however, preliminary discussion with the parents may very well set the tone of the diagnostic interview and even of any treatment that may follow.

It goes without saying that in those rare cases in which the youngster is suffering from too great a degree of intellectual retardation or emotional disturbance to be able to comprehend any explanation, the concern is only with getting the child to the psychiatrist's office.

Conducting the Interview

The entire clinical interview with the child should be conducted as an exploratory procedure. It is undertaken to obtain as clear a picture as possible of the reported or unreported difficulties.

Occasionally, a child who shares his parents' concern about one of his "problems" may invite some preliminary interpretation or suggestion for improving his functioning. But it is a good rule to refrain from making any attempts to change behavior during this initial session. Such efforts should be avoided not only because they would be premature, but also because any implied criticism of the child, especially if it can be interpreted as moralizing, tends to seal off opinions, resentments, hostility and apprehensions that require thorough investigation. This is true even if the youngster is giving an extremely distorted account of what has been going on around him. His own concepts of significant events and relationships in his life have to be brought to light and understood before one can begin to draw up any treatment plan for modifying these concepts.

One sometimes hears the opinion that diagnostic interviews with a child should not be highly structured, that his problems can be best evaluated if the sessions are permitted to move spontaneously. Naturally, the conduct of a specific interview will vary greatly in accordance with the child's age and other pertinent factors in his case, but a totally unstructured interview rarely, if ever, proves to be productive.

It has often been remarked that there will be as many different diagnoses of a child's condition as there are psychiatrists examining him. This complaint is partly due to the lack of comparability among the types of data on which many diagnostic formulations are based. Like the six blind men who touched different parts of the elephant's body, each diagnostician may have concentrated on a different facet of the child's behavior. Employment of a standard listing of items describing the mental status of children would go far toward remedying the difficulty. In the psychiatric diagnosis of an adult, an interview that did not follow a mental status schema would be regarded as inadequate. A diagnostic interview with a child should cover a group of similar items in the same consistent and comprehensive fashion. To be sure, the modes of communication through which the various items are explored have to be appropriate to the age of the child, and the items themselves have to be assessed in terms of the pertinent norms for age and sex.

Alerted by the history, the examiner can make a point of scrutinizing certain aspects of the child's functioning. The interview itself, as it progresses, will also make clear those items that justify lengthy and painstaking investigation and others that require only cursory observation. Coverage of the entire range of items is necessary, however, to insure the comparability and relevance of such diagnostic interviews.

The psychiatric interview should yield information on the following:

1. Spontaneous motility and speech.
2. Spontaneous choice of play material or topic of discussion.

3. Play performance and use of language.
4. Affective behavior (including the child's attitude toward the examiner.)
5. Stated interests and content of thought pertaining to them.
6. Attitudes toward family, school, and playmates, as reflected in the child's play productions or discussion.
7. The child's own evaluation of any problems specifically referred to in the history, or of any additional problems, such as fears or obsessions.
8. Temperamental characteristics.*

The first portion of the interview is devoted to putting the patient at ease and building up a positive relationship. As Kanner (1957) notes, the physician's first task is to help the child to sense acceptance, without giving him the impression of passivity and submissiveness: "The absence of irritation and a punitive attitude is not synonymous with inertia." With a preschool child, this relaxed atmosphere is usually achieved best by engaging him in the use of toys or play equipment.

To assure some form of pleasurable activity for children, the following basic equipment is suggested:

A play table.
A set of blocks.
Water colors, finger paints, crayons, plasticene, or clay.
Toy furnishings typifying a bedroom, bathroom, kitchen and schoolroom.
Puppets or dolls representing a father, mother, boy, girl and a baby; also figures of soldiers, cowboys, spacemen, etc.
A punching bag, dart guns and balloons.
Simple craft materials.

With an adolescent, and also with some preadolescents and even younger children, verbal interchange alone will pave the way to a

---

* Other clinicians have drawn up similar lists of functions to be evaluated in the interview. Shaw (1966), for example, suggests: (1) relationship capacity; (2) affect—especially anxiety, depression and anger; (3) intellectual capacity and intellectual functioning; (4) neurologic integration—motor, perceptual, conceptual; (5) reality-testing; (6) motivation; and (7) acculturation.

favorable relationship; for other youngsters, a combination of play and conversation may provide a better opening. If the child has been told that the psychiatrist would like to get to know him before advising his parents how best to help him with his problems, the session would logically open with a conversation on topics of positive interest to him.

A special approach is necessary in interviewing an adolescent who is in the throes of a hostile relationship with his parents. It may be advisable here to initiate the discussion of problems more directly. The psychiatrist might plunge immediately into the subject with a statement like the following: "I know that coming here today was really not your idea at all, but your parents are worried about the many fights going on at home (or about a teacher's complaints, or the youngster's coming in very late at night, or whatever the chief bone of contention may be). They have already told me what they think about it. I explained to them that I really could not be sure that I was giving the right suggestions if I heard only their side of the story and I asked them to let you come and tell me what you think about it. Anything you want to tell me will be private: it will not be repeated to your parents. Of course, it is up to you to decide whether anything can be gained by talking to me." When the psychiatrist makes clear that he has no intention of judging, berating or moralizing, even a very resentful youngster will often be able to relax and discuss his opinions and feelings in a meaningful way.

Outlining the Mental Status

Once the tone of the interview has been established, one can begin to study the patient's spontaneous motility and speech. These may fluctuate sharply, but any abnormalities in these areas will usually become manifest before the end of the interview.

Many a youngster will talk very freely, even to the point of becoming a chatterbox. However, one should distinguish between spontaneous activity and the production of a child who is making an obvious effort to be on his best behavior, perhaps by trying repeatedly to elicit clues to the examiner's preference in topics of discussion or play activity. Among many open-ended questions that may be asked are the following: What do you like to do best?

What would you like to be when you grow up? If you could do anything you wanted all day tomorrow, what would you do? The answers frequently lead to spontaneous discussions of dislikes and preferences. A child's choice of play material cannot be rated as spontaneous unless he is offered a wide range of possibilities. The fact that a child busies himself with crayons may not be significant if only graphic media are available to him. But the choice of such a quiet and sedentary activity as drawing may be revealing if the materials placed at his disposal permit diverse forms of play, among them such aggressive activities as punching or shooting.

A child who feels himself too old to "play with baby toys" and yet is too young to communicate solely through words may be encouraged to engage in some form of craft work. This may facilitate an evaluation of his ability to organize his thoughts and behavior; such activity may also reveal the degree of self-confidence and creativity he possesses or highlight such issues as dependency, negativism or good comradeship. Putting a child's hands to work may also make it possible for him to be less self-conscious in his verbal communications.

To be of value, the description of the child's play and verbal communications must be specifically assessed in terms of their level and content for one in his own age group. Simple repetitive play or talk by a tot who has just passed his second birthday would have absolutely no pathologic significance, whereas such activity in a ten year old would warrant close examination. The form and content of the child's production may reveal the presence of gross pathology, or may throw light on the child's interpersonal relationships, his reactions to the success or failure of his endeavors, and his concept of himself.

The affective components of behavior can be assessed as a youngster plays, does craft work, talks, or withdraws from activity. In the course of an interview, a continuous change in affect may be observed. If, after manifesting a restrained, shy and apprehensive manner, a child becomes progressively more at ease during the interview, so that he appears relaxed and spontaneous when it ends, one should explore several possibilities. Was his initial conduct typical of his reactions to a new situation? If so, is this due to a temperamental pattern and essentially an expression of normalcy?

Or is it an excessive reaction indicating pathology? If the child has only recently manifested this apprehensive reaction to new situations, what specific events account for the change? In some children, on the other hand, there appears to be an instant trust and intimacy, as if they had known the examiner all their lives. This pattern too may justify investigation. Again, one may ask if the behavior represents a normal temperamental reaction or pathology.

Evidence of hostile attitudes, depressed feelings, tenseness and anxiety ought also to be explored in the diagnostic interview.

The child's stated interests and their elaboration may be pertinent to problems referred to in the history or may appear to be far removed from them. Many children are not aware of those aspects of their functioning that alarm their parents. Some youngsters, however, may be greatly concerned over difficulties about which their parents have no knowledge or to which they have given only scant recognition. The psychiatrist should avoid plunging too quickly into the problems described in the history, for he might thereby lose the opportunity to investigate other preoccupations and worries that the child finds it difficult to discuss.

Whenever possible, one should elicit the child's own statement of his adaptation. His view of the areas considered to be problems by his parents and others is an important part of judging the child's reality-testing and capacity for changing attitudes and behavior. Often, once one asks a child what his concerns are, he may bring up problems that have not been mentioned before. He may welcome the chance to discuss them with an uninvolved person. In fact, it may even turn out that the new issues he introduces will form the major portion of the interview.

The child's own evaluation of his parents, siblings, teachers and playmates, and of the quality of their relationship to him, represents another area of investigation. If he is very young, this information may be elicited through the content of his play; otherwise, it may be more easily obtained through discussion. One may get truer responses indirectly by chatting about an area of relationship than would be forthcoming through the question-answer routine. Too many children appear to have trained themselves to give, as they would in school, "proper" answers to questions rather than to divulge what they really think. A discussion of the nuisance value of little brothers may yield more data on sibling relationships than a direct inquiry would produce.

Clinical Observation of Temperament

Observations of the child's behavior during a clinical play interview can supply useful information on the child's temperamental attributes, some of which may have a direct bearing on his behavior problem.

Whatever the setting, a child will show characteristics of his own behavioral style. But the specific setting and its meaning to the child will also influence his activity, helping to determine whether it is boisterous or quiet, adventurous or timid, gay or fearful, high speed or low. If a three year old in the examiner's office sticks close to his mother's skirts and cannot be coaxed into talking, this may in part be because he is afraid of the doctor, but may also reflect a characteristic reaction to a new situation.

To what extent is behavior observed in an artificial setting typical of a child? This pertinent question has been raised most cogently by Freeman (1967). He emphasizes that the office observation may not be a representative sampling of the child's reaction style for several reasons: (1) It is a specialized setting with connotations that may influence the youngster's behavior. To a child who attends nursery school, the playroom with its blocks, trucks and dolls may invoke toy usage that reflects his adaptation to a permissive nursery setting but may give little information about his behavior in routine home activities. (2) The one-to-one child-observer format fails to give a picture of the patient's interaction with other children. In a pediatric or psychiatric clinic, a play group is sometimes available, and the observation can then include interactions with other children in either a free play or a structured situation. (3) The stimuli are relatively limited and hence we do not have the opportunity to see how the youngster reacts to the many competing stimuli of the school or home setting, which may indeed be the focus of the presenting complaints. (4) The office observation necessarily comprises a limited time span, and some aspects of temperamental reactivity may not be demonstrable by definition—for example, persistence of an extraordinary degree. (5) The child may react to the unfamiliarity of the office with behavior that reflects one side of his reactive style. He may be subdued or more hopped up; he may be on his best behavior or his worst.

Despite these limitations, one can usually obtain useful data about temperamental expressivity during an office observation.

Activity Level

This may manifest itself in two ways: the speed with which a child carries out an individual act and the frequency with which he shifts from one activity to another. The highly active child draws a picture with hasty strokes, throws darts rapidly, runs rather than walks. He may also move from one fast action to another with no rest periods in between. In general, he will appear to move more quickly or shift his activity more often than the average child of his age.

Intensity of Reaction

Does the child express pleasure exuberantly, or can only a bare smile be coaxed out of him? Is he loud when he fusses or does pain or movement restriction result merely in a whine? Some children exhibit an intermediate degree of intensity, while others manifest varying degrees in their intensity of reaction, depending on the specific events occurring during the observation.

Quality of Mood

An observer can attempt to estimate the proportion of time in which positive and negative moods are expressed by the child. Here one notes the deviation from neutral mood in the one or other direction, without consideration of the vigor or gentleness with which its presence is made known.

Approach or Withdrawal

The youngster who must be restrained from exploring the office, strikes up conversations, and is interested immediately in everything and everybody is clearly a high approacher. One may easily identify the high withdrawer as the child who won't initially be separated from parents, barely answers questions, shows little interest in office toys though he may play with those he has brought from home. Other children show more moderate reactions.

Adaptability

The withdrawing youngster who becomes more at home within a half hour to an hour, who moves from silence to chattering, from abstainer to extensive toy user, has a high adaptability. Indeed, when such a youngster warms up he may appear to be a highly active and intense child and one may wish for a formula to cool him down somewhat. Long-term adaptability cannot, of course, be identified in a single observation. One may gain some knowledge of this characteristic if the child remains in the hospital for several weeks, or if a number of observations are made in the same setting spaced over weeks or even months.

Threshold of Responsiveness

This may be difficult to note in the office unless it is unusually high or low. One may nevertheless be able to note the youngster with hyperacuity of auditory, visual, tactile, olfactory and pain awareness. Some youngsters, while sensorily intact, seem to require a high level of stimulation before responding.

Distractibility

A child's response to the competing stimuli of many toys in the observer's office may indicate the level of his distractibility. His attention may be pulled away from his ongoing activity with blocks by the punching bag, the dart board or a puppet. If he continually shifts his full attention to each object that should ordinarily have been noted or mentioned in passing, one may reasonably conclude that he has a high degree of distractibility. In the usual psychiatric office playroom, there is no opportunity to note the degree of distractibility stimulated by the presence of many different persons in the environment. However, if the observation is done in a pediatric clinic, there will be many other children and the degree of distractibility may be more fully assessed.

Attention Span and Persistence

The comments on distractibility are also pertinent here. If the child has become engrossed in an activity appropriate to his age or to his specific interest, his continued involvement despite competing stimuli, or his ability to return to the activity after distraction, may indicate his attention span and persistence. On the other hand, if he is apprehensive about an impending medical procedure or if appropriate materials to elicit interest are not available, one may not be able to ascertain his typical behavior. Under ideal observational circumstances, one may be able to determine whether the child has long or short attention span, high or low persistence with regard to activities and social interchange. A child may have high persistence in pursuing an interpersonal relationship and low persistence in task pursuit, and the reverse may also be true.

Number of Interviews

In most cases, a single diagnostic interview will be adequate, but more than one session may be required if the youngster is so frightened or hostile that he refuses to talk or cooperate during the first visit. Sometimes half of the session may be taken up in persuading a youngster to enter the playroom. Children are often fearful because parents have informed them about the visit in a threatening manner. A youngster may resist the interview because he sees it as proof that he is "wicked" or "crazy." Trouble may also result if the parents have been dishonest in explaining the purpose of the visit—for example, if they told the child he was merely accompanying mother "to the doctor."

Under such circumstances the initial interview may be quite unproductive, although it does provide the psychiatrist with an opportunity to establish the fact that he is not an ogre and that he has some playthings in his office that a youngster would enjoy using.

When special difficulties are encountered, it may be necessary to conduct a series of sessions devoted to diagnostic study. By and large, however, the psychiatrist has a responsibility to formulate a basic diagnosis as early as possible, so that a treatment program can be promptly planned and instituted.

Family Diagnosis

A current trend in child psychiatry is the emphasis on gathering the entire family to participate in the diagnostic interview. The rationale for this procedure is that the child's behavior can be best understood in the context of his interaction with the family group.

Among the leading proponents of this view are Ackerman (1958) and Williams (1968), who contend that the group session enables the psychiatrist to observe in living terms how the family interactions precipitate certain intrapsychic patterns in the child. The investigators point out that many nonverbal instructions, encouraging transgressions that are avowedly deplored, may not be seen in the classical diagnostic workup but may appear with great clarity in a family setting.

It is also maintained that a child who feels guilty about "talking behind my parents' back" will speak more freely when the parents are present. Presumably, too, the group session protects the child's self-esteem; since the family becomes the "patient," the youngster is spared being singled out as the "nut." An undercurrent of marital conflict may also become apparent in the family session, perhaps revealing that the parents use the child as a scapegoat to avoid recognition of their own problem.

In certain instances, there is merit in the idea of bringing together the entire family or selected members for diagnostic purposes. This was advocated by some child psychiatrists before family diagnosis became an institutionalized procedure. Allen (1963), for example, in his many years of work with the Philadelphia Child Guidance Clinic, found it essential to consider the family as a unit in the diagnostic process.

In my own practice, I have assumed that both parents should be seen in the sessions devoted to history-taking and discussion of recommendations. In the diagnostic interview, I have seen the child either alone, together with one or both parents, or one or more sibs, as seemed most productive. The principle of selectivity is of first importance. I would question the family diagnosis as a routine procedure in all cases. Either the individual or the family diagnostic session may be appropriate, depending on the circumstances: the specific child, family and behavior problem that may be involved.

For example, let us assume the history indicates that a mother finds her child unmanageable, and that the father subtly encourages this problem. It does not automatically follow that the child should be seen together with his parents in order to reenact this relationship. On the contrary, it may be more useful to find out how the child behaves in a situation structured by the dignostician. Examining the pattern of the child's behavior in the presence of his parents is not the be-all and end-all of diagnosis. While some children may talk more freely when their parents are in the room, others are more inhibited. In some cases it may be desirable to have both types of diagnostic session: one with the child alone, and a second in the family setting. The psychiatrist should be flexible and selective in his approach. His decision should be governed not by a rigid theoretic formula but by the nature of the living problem at hand.

SELECTED REFERENCES

Ackerman, N. W.: *The Psychodynamics of Family Life.* New York, Basic Books, 1958.
Allen, F. H.: *Positive Aspects of Child Psychiatry.* New York, W. W. Norton, 1963.
Freeman, R.: The home visit in child psychiatry: Its usefulness in diagnosis and training. *J. Amer. Acad. Child Psychiat.* 6:276-294, 1967.
Group for the Advancement of Psychiatry: *The Diagnostic Process in Child Psychiatry.* New York, Group for the Advancement of Psychiatry, Report No. 38, 1957.
Kanner, L.: *Child Psychiatry.* Springfield, Ill., Charles C Thomas, 1957.
McDonald, M.: The psychiatric evaluation of children. *J. Amer. Acad. Child Psychiat.* 4:569-612, 1965.
Shaw, C. R.: *The Psychiatric Disorders of Childhood.* New York, Appleton-Century-Crofts, 1966.
Sullivan, H. S.: *The Psychiatric Interview.* New York, W. W. Norton, 1954.
Williams, F. S.: Family therapy. *In* Marmor, J. (Ed.): *Modern Psychoanalysis.* New York, Basic Books, 1968.
Yarrow, L. J.: Interviewing children. *In* Mussen, P. H. (Ed.): *Handbook of Research Methods in Child Development.* New York, Wiley, 1960.

7. Special Diagnostic Procedures

To CLARIFY THE DIAGNOSTIC PICTURE developed in the history and direct interview, the psychiatrist may require additional data. At this point, he finds it helpful to make use of special fact-finding procedures. He may call upon a psychologist to conduct various tests, or he may consult a neurologist or other medical specialist. In rare instances, the use of inpatient facilities will be indicated to complete the diagnostic formulation.

Psychologic Procedures

Usually, the questions to be asked of the psychologist arise from information obtained in both the history and psychiatric interview. In some cases, however, the history reveals areas of uncertainty in which specific psychologic data could be helpful before the child is seen.

The psychologist may be asked to evaluate the child's level of intelligence by administering one or another type of psychometric examination. He may also examine special aspects of personality development through an interpretation of the child's responses to an organized group of materials.

To administer a full battery of psychologic tests to every child being diagnosed would be as much out of order as it would be to request a full series of gastrointestinal x-rays for every patient complaining of a stomachache. Like the diagnostic procedures at the command of the medical practitioner, psychologic tests have to be used with selectivity to obtain specific information.

Since individual judgment and other subjective factors affect the scoring systems of these supplementary diagnostic procedures, especially in the projective techniques, the choice of examiner is not to be regarded as a routine consideration. Not all psychologists are equally equipped to deal with children. Skill in putting children at their ease is required, as well as a knowledge of the criteria to be employed in evaluating a child's performance or appraising his personality. If, for example, a psychologist who is accustomed to reading the Rorschach responses of adults interpreted the responses of a five or six year old by the same standards, he would find indications of abnormality in certain reactions that are actually normal for a young subject. For proper evaluation, each procedure requires a thorough understanding of the capacities and characteristics of children at every age level.

The preparation of a child who is to be referred for testing and the selection of an appropriate time are other matters that require attention. Since a child's vitality and state of mind can affect his performance on a test, he should be told about the forthcoming procedure in a manner most likely to mobilize his best effort. A very young child, for instance, might be most receptive to the idea that he was being invited to work on some puzzles or to play a few games. If the child has not completely recovered from an illness or the effects of some emotionally charged experience, it is better to postpone the testing than to run the risk that the results will not reflect the youngster's characteristic performance.

Some of the tests, notably those measuring intelligence, are available in group as well as in individual form, but the testing of children in groups is not generally recommended for purposes of individual diagnosis. In a group, there is a greater likelihood that a youngster may misunderstand directions and that he may be adversely affected by the tension of the situation itself. Moreover, since children being tested together may yield to the temptation to copy answers from one another, their scores may be tipped to their own advantage or disadvantage. Individual testing enables the psychologist to observe situational factors that may prevent a child from achieving his optimum score, and this may sometimes be the most valuable finding. The examiner who deals with one child at a time also has a greater opportunity to create a relaxed and friendly atmosphere before proceeding with the formal testing.

In making use of the various psychologic tests, the child psychiatrist must be fully aware of their values and limitations. Each procedure has to be regarded as a laboratory instrument; its results are to be viewed not in isolation but as part of a pattern of behavior. One should bear in mind that none of the projective tests has ever been completely validated. It would, indeed, be impossible to validate some of the procedures, but even those which might be statistically evaluated have not been subjected to rigorous predictive testing. Moreover, since the results in part reflect the interpretive skill of the examiner, the same test administered to a child by different psychologists or on different occasions by the same psychologist can lead to varying findings.

All the testing procedures are more or less culture-bound, with experiential factors playing a role in the subject's performance. Intelligence quotients on tests that have proved to be generally reliable for groups of middle-class white youngsters living in cities in the northeastern part of the United States are biased for similar groups living in the southern part of the country or in rural areas, for those whose families are in lower income brackets, or for nonwhite youngsters. To overcome the more obvious limitations of the tests, special versions have been prepared for various language or geographic groups. Nevertheless, none of these special examinations merits unqualified acceptance.

One of the chief values of these supplementary diagnostic procedures is that they enable the psychiatrist to confirm the existence of certain mental attitudes that were not clearly delineated during the diagnostic interview. The tests help the psychiatrist differentiate between disorganized and well-organized functioning and between mental dependency and independence; he also can determine on the basis of relatively objective data whether his subject is overestimating his personal capacities or has a realistic view of himself. In the course of formal testing, too, any unusual ability to conceptualize or to persevere in a task is almost certain to manifest itself. Quick changes of mood and any exceptional sensitivity to the examiner or to particular sights and sounds will emerge distinctly. Evidences of hyperactivity, short attention span, distractibility, perseveration, compulsive behavior or obsessive thinking also come into clear focus.

If, as occasionally happens, a child's test performance is strikingly inconsistent with the history and clinical picture, neither type of evidence should be rejected in favor of the other. A thorough study of the apparently contradictory findings will usually yield an explanation that enhances the diagnostician's understanding of the young patient's problems. A determined effort to resolve such a discrepancy may uncover facts that are pivotal.

If tests given under the most favorable conditions yield scores higher than those reflected in the child's report cards, this does not necessarily signify that he can do equally well in his schoolwork. A substantial difference in performance would suggest, rather, that some of the child's reactions to the school situation merit further investigation and might well serve as a focus of individual treatment or environmental manipulation.

Another possible reason for contradictory findings is that the permissive atmosphere of the diagnostic interview stimulates one pattern of behavior, while the formality of the test situation sparks a quite different type of conduct. Differences in the sexual and racial identities of the two examiners, in their personal appearance, or in their approach to the youngster may influence his responses, thus providing clues to significant psychopathology.

The psychologist administering a diagnostic test should be briefed on its precise purpose. He should have some knowledge of the youngster's difficulties, any suspected pathology, and the aspects of functioning that the psychiatrist is trying to clarify. For example, the tester should be informed that a child is being examined to determine whether some of his learning difficulties are due to perceptual defects rather than to mental retardation.

The psychologic procedures most often used as diagnostic aids in child psychiatry fall into four major categories: intelligence tests, achievement tests, special clinical explorations of impairments in functioning, and projective techniques. Each of these procedures will be briefly discussed.

Intelligence Tests

When the need arises to check the clinical impressions of a youngster's intellectual ability, an intelligence test is in order. Among the tests most often given are the Stanford-Binet test and the Wechsler Intelligence Scale for Children (WISC). Special tests for preschool children include the Cattell Infant Intelligence Scale, the Wechsler Preschool and Primary Scale of Intelligence (WPPSI), and the Gesell Developmental Schedules. For adolescents, the Wechsler Adult Intelligence Scale (WAIS) is also employed.

The psychologist who gives one of these tests is expected to provide the child psychiatrist with findings that go beyond the numerical score. Some commentary on the applicability of the test results to the subject's general level of intellectual functioning is needed. In addition to the score, the report should indicate the basal mental age and ceiling of intelligence; these represent respectively the highest mental age at which the child can answer all the test items and that at which he can answer none of the items. When the test is used for diagnostic purposes, information is also needed on any variability in subtest results, as well as on any marked inconsistencies or discrepancies in performance. In addition, the psychologist may often provide information about the child's individual way of handling the tests.

The psychologist's observations about any anxiety, distress or other attitudes manifested by the child during the test are highly relevant, since the diagnostician wants to know if the situation stimulated the youngster's most efficient functioning or held him back. The examiner should also specify whether the intellectual functioning of his subject is even or uneven, and in the event it is uneven, whether it reflects a consistent pattern of ability or disability in a given area. Notations on any marked disturbances in the child's attention span or on an easy distractibility which may have interfered with his test performance are also helpful to the psychiatrist.

However, evidence of anxiety about certain areas of functioning covered in an examination does not invariably account for low scores. Inability to perform well, though often attributed to anxiety while dealing with particular subjects, may represent a true index of intellectual capacity. Hence, while it is important to note any signs of uneasiness evoked by specific aspects of a testing procedure, it is essential to determine whether a child's anxieties actually influenced his execution or merely reflected an awareness of his limitations in a given area of mental functioning.

Achievement Tests

Achievement tests may enter into the diagnostic process when the psychiatrist wishes to determine whether a youngster has benefited from his schooling to the degree to be expected, or whether he is educationally advanced or retarded. Various types of standard scholastic tests have been devised to indicate the grade level achieved by the subject.

One of the more commonly used procedures is the Wide Range Achievement Test, which can be administered to children five years of age or older. Another is the Metropolitan Achievement Test, which contains batteries of material for school children in grades one through eight. The Iowa High School Test, the Stanford Achievement Test, and the Gates Reading Test are also used frequently for diagnostic purposes.

Some of these tests are designed to gauge achievement in a single area, such as reading facility. Others cover a range of subjects.

Special Clinical Tests

Certain techniques are employed to test impaired functioning in cases of cerebral dysfunction and for other special purposes. In this category are the Bender Visual Motor Gestalt Test and the Goldstein-Scheerer Tests.

The Bender Visual Motor Gestalt Test calls for the reproduction of geometric forms or designs which differ in their complexity and relationships to one another. The accuracy of the reproduction varies normally in accordance with the age of the child being tested. Marked deviations in his performance from that expected at his age level may be of considerable significance. Some characteristic distortions in the reproduced designs may point to perceptual defects or difficulty in hand-eye coordination, while others suggest functional disorders or inability to concentrate.

The Goldstein-Scheerer Tests have been designed to provide both quantitative and qualitative measurements of the reasoning ability of patients suffering from brain damage. The subject's ability to deal with both abstract and concrete concepts is evaluated through these procedures.

Projective Tests

Projective techniques are used to obtain fuller information about a child's personality and his relationships, whether to the world in general or to specific figures in it. Among the procedures frequently employed for this purpose are the Rorschach Test, the Thematic Apperception Test, and the Goodenough Draw-a-Man Test.

The Rorschach Test materials consist of a series of cards with inkblots of symmetric design. One by one, in a designated order, these cards are presented to the child, who is asked to describe what he sees in the blots. Human beings, animals, landscapes and inanimate objects are usually visualized, in whole or in part, in movement or motionless, with good or poor perception of the forms, colors or shadings appearing in the test figures. Abnormal perceptions and preoccupations may often be discerned by analyzing a child's responses and comparing them with those most commonly given.

The Thematic Apperception Test (TAT) and related procedures such as the Children's Apperception Test (CAT) and the Blacky Test are also conducted with sets of cards. Each card in the first test depicts a scene with one or more persons while the cards used for the CAT and Blacky Test portray animals. The scenes, though suggestive of activities, are vague enough to permit a wide range of interpretations of the actions or moods of the figures presented. The child is asked to describe the scene and to complete the story it suggests. His narrative frequently contains clues to his impressions of his relations with significant figures in his environment, to areas in which his perceptions are consistently distorted, and to particular preoccupations or deviant modes of thought.

The Goodenough Draw-a-Man Test, as its name suggests, focuses on the drawing of a human figure. The subject is graded on his ability to delineate parts of the body and is given additional points for the correctness of their placement and proportioning in relation to one another. Mental age is determined on the basis of the total number of points received. Since there is a high degree of correlation between these scores and those achieved on intelligence tests, especially with respect to items that are considered to tap "social intelligence," the Draw-a-Man Test is often used as an instrument for measuring intelligence quickly. For many children with cerebral dysfunction, particularly postencephalitic behavior disorder, or for those with sociopathic personalities, the Goodenough score falls significantly below that for the complete intelligence test. The drawings of subjects suffering from childhood schizophrenia or certain types of organic brain disorders often point to distorted perceptions, especially when the human figure is drawn in a fragmented way or when the emphasis placed on one or another anatomic detail is much greater than is to be expected of a child in the subject's age group. Because the child's drawing does not bear a one-to-one relationship to his overall psychiatric status, one should be wary of coming to conclusions based solely on drawings.

Projective-test responses have to be interpreted with particular caution. Some that appear highly pathologic may be accurate representations of experiences which happen to be outside the ken of the examiner. For example, the responses of two sisters on the Rorschach and Thematic Apperception tests showed repetitive percepts of violent altercations taking place between persons who fell asleep in the midst of battle so that the pictured conflict never reached the point of resolution. Clinically, however, the little girls appeared to be normal. Subsequent investigation revealed that their test responses conveyed an accurate impression of their life. Their parents actually did fight violently, but in the midst of these battles, the mother would retire to bed and remain there sleeping for several days. Long-term observation of the sisters confirmed their intrinsic normalcy.

Medical Consultations

Information obtained in the course of history-taking or the initial face-to-face study of the child may prompt the diagnostician to investigate the possible physiologic origins of a behavior disorder or, on the other hand, to confirm the presumably psychogenic nature of certain physical symptoms.

When the existence of neurologic damage is suspected, a neurologic examination and an electroencephalogram of a child will provide valuable information. To insure their adequacy and accuracy, these procedures should be performed by a physician who has learned the special techniques required for the neurologic examination of children. He must also be able to gain their cooperation. Otherwise a youngster under examination may become so frightened that his refusal to cooperate or his muscular tension will make it difficult, if not impossible, to obtain accurate findings.

The testing of postural reflexes and other aspects of immature nervous functioning that do not ordinarily figure in the neurologic examination of adults may uncover important signs of pathology in a young child. Moreover, since the electroencephalogram of a child differs from that of an adult, its proper interpretation depends on knowledge of what is normal for different periods of childhood. These considerations justify particular care in the selection of the neurologist to be consulted, and also explain why the practice of pediatric neurology is now regarded as a subspeciality in the field of neurology.

Consultations with other specialists are not infrequently required to help resolve diagnostic uncertainties. Auditory tests are essential to determine whether partial deafness may be contributing to mental retardation, learning difficulties or a behavior disorder. Ophthalmologic examination is indicated when poor vision is suspected of being a contributing factor. To decide whether an endocrine study should be conducted in a case, consultation with a pediatrician may be warranted. Orthopedic or hematologic consultation also may be indicated for the purpose of fitting together a total picture.

When parents have assumed that a physical symptom is emotionally determined and when this is not at all clear, the opinion of the appropriate consultant will help the psychiatrist to identify the true significance of the symptom. For example, the parents of one child were reluctant to believe that his asthma was not psychogenic. However, the results of an examination by an allergist convinced them that the malady was in fact due to a specific allergy. The sudden tendency of a little girl to cling to her mother at a time when the girl's baby brother was learning to walk was attributed to sibling rivalry by her mother, but the orthopedist who was called into consultation confirmed the psychiatrist's suspicion that the child's dependent behavior was caused by a disease that was producing progressive muscular weakness.

Use of Inpatient Facilities

In a small number of cases, differential diagnosis is so complicated and difficult that it seems virtually impossible to complete the diagnosis while the child remains at home. If, for example, the parents' descriptions of their child's current behavior appear to be grossly unreliable, or if their own behavior or some traumatic situation in the home appears to be the major cause of his psychopathology, it may be important to observe how the child behaves in a controlled situation. Hospital observation may also be indicated if his symptoms spell out danger to himself or those around him. The failure of a treatment plan already instituted may point to the need for a more adequate trial of the measures recommended, or for a reevaluation of the diagnostic understanding upon which the plan was based.

Inpatient diagnostic facilities for children are much scarcer and more costly than equivalent facilities for adults. Proper observation of a child requires a residential set-up approximating his normal daily routine—that is, one with school and recreational facilities as well as with the usual provisions for physical care and detailed psychiatric study. Since some private sanatoria and public hospitals, though generally ill-equipped to observe younger children properly, have diagnostic units for adolescents or will accommodate them on the adult wards, the shortage of facilities is less serious for the teen-ager than for younger patients. An expansion of the now meager inpatient diagnostic facilities for children as well as for adults is anticipated in view of the trend toward the establishment of psychiatric wards in general hospitals.

SELECTED REFERENCES

Anastasi, A.: *Psychological Testing.* 3rd edition. New York, Macmillan, 1968.
Anderson, H. H., and Anderson, G. L. (Eds.): *An Introduction to Projective Techniques and Other Devices for Understanding the Dynamics of Human Behavior.* New York, Prentice-Hall, 1951.
Bender, L.: *A Visual Motor Gestalt Test and Its Clinical Use.* Research Monograph No. 3. New York, American Orthopsychiatric Association, 1938.
Terman, L. M., and Merrill, M. A.: *Revised Stanford-Binet Intelligence Scale.* Boston, Houghton Mifflin, 1960.
Tyler, L. E.: *The Psychology of Human Differences.* New York, Appleton-Century-Crofts, 1965.

8. Diagnostic Classification

THE STANDARDIZATION of diagnostic terms in child psychiatry presents a difficult problem. Various schools of thought, training centers, and individual psychiatrists have a tendency to use diagnostic tags that reflect their own theoretic concepts. For example the term "pregenital behavior disorder" is based on a presupposition that is not universally accepted. A diagnosis of disturbance in the parent-child relationship may express only the clinician's idea of faulty interpersonal relationships. To complicate things, there is no general agreement on whether the diagnostic nomenclature should be based on etiology, presenting symptoms, prognosis, or a combination of these factors.

An additional difficulty is noted by Kolb (1968), who observes that "Since there is less fixity of the patterns of disturbed behavior because of the plastic personality of the child, there is less unanimity in regard to the diagnostic schemata for the disorders of childhood than for those of adulthood." Shaw (1966) agrees with this author that one of the vexing aspects of diagnosis in disturbed children is their propensity for change—in symptoms as well as personality— as they grow up.

Some child psychiatrists believe that behavioral pathology should be classified by phenomenologic groupings, such as antisocial behavior, habit disorders and phobias. This descriptive approach, which categorizes symptoms manifested by the child, has been criticized on two main grounds: (1) there is no necessary correlation between symptom and disease; and (2) the emphasis on differences in manifest symptomatology neglects underlying pathogenic factors. Anna Freud (1965), for example, maintains that symptoms in childhood, unlike comparable ones in adults, may be produced nonpathologically by stresses and strains inherent in development itself. She defines average development norms for all aspects of personality, and bases the diagnosis on a child's deviance from these norms.

In the United States, the most authoritative guide to diagnostic nomenclature for patients of all ages is the *Diagnostic and Statis-*

97

tical Manual of Mental Disorders, issued by the American Psychiatric Association. Initially published in 1952, this manual was extensively revised in 1968. Since it is based on a wide consensus and has official recognition, the APA classification facilitates statistical coding of comparable data from various sources. In its revised form, the manual also represents an advance toward the use of a standard international classification system. It attempts, so far as possible, to coordinate American terminology with that of the World Health Organization's *International Classification of Diseases* (1968).

The APA's diagnostic nomenclature is divided into ten major sections, each containing a number of subdivisions. Following is a list of the categories, with brief comments on those most relevant to childhood disorders.

1. *Mental Retardation.* In the 1952 edition of the APA manual, this category was called "mental deficiency" and placed last. The shift in terminology and position is significant. Formerly, only the idiopathic or familial types of retardation were included. When the disorder was due to a chronic brain syndrome, it was classified as a chronic brain syndrome "with mental deficiency." Now, however, mental retardation is placed first to emphasize that the condition is to be diagnosed whenever present, even if due to some other disorder. New ways of thinking about the causes of mental retardation are also reflected in two subsections: retardation "following major psychiatric disorder" and "with psycho-social (environmental) deprivation." (For a detailed classification of mental retardation, see chapter 9 of this volume.)

2. *Organic Brain Syndromes.* These syndromes are grouped into psychotic and nonpsychotic disorders according to the severity of functional impairment. "The severity of the associated symptoms is affected by and related to not only the precipitating organic disorder but also the patient's inherent personality patterns, present emotional conflicts, his environmental situation, and interpersonal relations."

3. *Psychoses Not Attributed to Physical Conditions Listed Previously.* This category includes schizophrenia, affective disorders, paranoid states and other psychoses. There is a subclassification for schizophrenia of the childhood type.

4. *Neuroses.*

5. *Personality Disorders and Certain Other Nonpsychotic Mental Disorders.*

6. *Psychophysiologic Disorders.* This deals with physical disorders of presumably psychogenic origin.

7. *Special symptoms.* This category includes speech disturbance, specific learning disturbance, tic, disorder of sleep, feeding disturbance and enuresis.

8. *Transient Situational Disturbances.* Included in this group are "more or less transient disorders of any severity (including those of psychotic proportions) that occur in individuals without any apparent underlying disorders and that represent an acute reaction to overwhelming environmental stress. A diagnosis in this category should specify the cause and manifestations of the disturbance so far as possible. If the patient has good adaptive capacity his symptoms usually recede as the stress diminishes. If, however, the symptoms persist after the stress is removed, the diagnosis of another mental disorder is indicated." Disorders are classified according to the patient's developmental stage, and include adjustment reaction of infancy, such as grief reaction associated with separation from patient's mother; adjustment reaction of childhood, such as jealousy associated with the birth of patient's younger sibling; and adjustment reaction of adolescence, such as irritability and depression associated with school failure and manifested by temper outbursts, brooding and discouragement.

9. *Behavior Disorders of Childhood and Adolescence.* This category embraces disorders that are more stable, internalized and resistant to treatment than transient situational disturbances, but less so than psychoses, neuroses and personality disorders. "This intermediate stability is attributed to the greater fluidity of all behavior at this age. Characteristic manifestations include such symptoms as overactivity, inattentiveness, shyness, feeling of rejection, over-aggressiveness, timidity, and delinquency." The following subdivisions of childhood and adolescent behavior disorders are presented:

Hyperkinetic reaction. ("If this behavior is caused by organic brain damage, it should be diagnosed under the appropriate nonpsychotic organic brain syndrome.")

Withdrawing reaction. ("This diagnosis should be reserved for those who cannot be classified as having schizophrenia and whose tendencies toward withdrawal have not yet stabilized enough to justify the diagnosis of schizoid personality.")
Overanxious reaction. This is to be distinguished from neurosis.
Runaway reaction.
Unsocialized aggressive reaction.
Group delinquent reaction.

10. *Conditions Without Manifest Psychiatric Disorder and Nonspecific Conditions.* Most of the subcategories under this heading—such as marital or occupational maladjustment—do not apply to children; however, cases of juvenile delinquency without discernible psychiatric disorder come under this heading.

Since individuals may have more than one mental disorder, a classification scheme must make room for multiple psychiatric diagnoses. Thus, there are children whose disorders could be diagnosed as both "Schizophrenia, childhood type" and "Mental retardation following major psychiatric disorder." However, as the APA manual emphasizes, the psychiatrist should observe the rule of parsimony and avoid diagnosing more conditions than are necessary to account for the clinical picture. "The opportunity to make multiple diagnoses does not lessen the physician's responsibility to make a careful differential diagnosis."

In deciding which of several diagnoses to list first, the psychiatrist uses his own judgment. He may find it advisable to list first the condition most urgently requiring treatment; if treatment priority is not an issue, the more serious condition should be listed first. The APA manual recommends that the diagnostician underscore on the patient's record the disorder he considers the underlying one. It is also recommended that associated physical conditions, when known, should be indicated in addition to the diagnosis of the mental disorder.

A classification system for psychopathologic disorders in childhood was formulated by the Group for the Advancement of Psychiatry in 1966, based on a theoretic framework that includes the psychosomatic concept, the developmental dimension and the psychosocial aspects of the child's existence. Disorders are arranged in a hierarchy of ten major categories, starting with healthy responses, proceeding through milder to more severe psychologic disorders, and then to syndromes in which somatic factors predominate. The following categories are proposed: (1) healthy responses, (2) reactive disorders, (3) developmental deviations, (4) psychoneurotic disorders, (5) personality disorders, (6) psychotic disorders, (7) psychophysiologic disorders, (8) brain syndromes, (9) mental retardation, and (10) other disorders.

For practical clinical purposes, a simplified diagnostic classification is often helpful. In my own practice, I have found it advantageous to use the following groupings: (1) normal, (2) mental retardation, (3) organic brain disturbance, (4) reactive behavior disorders, (5) neurotic behavior disorders, (6) neurotic character disorders, (7) neurosis, (8) childhood psychosis and schizophrenic adjustments, and (9) sociopathic personality. These categories have proved useful both in formulating etiology and in planning therapy. A brief characterization of each group follows. More detailed discussions appear in later chapters.

Normal

The fact that a child is brought to a psychiatrist for study does not necessarily mean, of course, that a psychologic disturbance is present. One function of the diagnostic process is to identify the normal child who has come to psychiatric notice because his behavior has been incorrectly interpreted. Parents or various referral sources may have faulty notions about norms of behavior and intellectual capacity. Or a child may be undergoing a minor maturational stress, not sufficiently severe to be classified as a psychiatric illness.

Unfortunately, obtaining agreement about the definition of normalcy in behavior is even more difficult than obtaining agreement on the definition of pathologic entities. As a working concept, keeping in mind its subjective nature, one may identify the following broad characteristics of a normal child: He gets along reasonably well with parents, siblings and friends; has few overt manifestations of behavioral disturbance; is using his apparent intellectual potential to approximate capacity; and is contented a reasonable proportion of the time.

This description covers a wide range of temperamental and personality patterns, extending from the somewhat shy to the somewhat aggressive child, from the quiet to the active type, from the individual whose threshold of tolerance to sensation and frustration is low to one with a high threshold, from the child with intense reactivity to one with quiet reactivity, from the child with a short attention span to one with a long attention span. In our society, we have a habit of conceptualizing as the "normal" personality a nonexistent "All-American Child" who is outgoing, athletic, gregarious and enthusiastic. This stereotype often results in labeling some youngsters as "problem children" simply because they deviate from this so-called norm. The shy child is often assumed to be fearful when he is, in line with his personality, merely cautious or reserved. One should not arbitrarily consider certain children as abnormal because their conduct is identified with types of behavior that do not conform to an abstraction. The range of normal behavior patterns is much wider than is generally believed. Of course, any extreme attributes of personality, in interaction with the environment, may assume a pathologic form.

Mental Retardation

The study of mental retardation, despite some noteworthy early work, was long the stepchild of psychiatry. In recent years, however, there has been a resurgence of interest in retarded children and the detailed dynamics of their behavior.

The retardate has a set of problems constantly related to his slowness of intellectual development. These problems are far from simple and require differentiated study. Many retarded youngsters present no actual behavior problems; the only issues that arise are those of appropriate management. However, behavior disorders occur with greater frequency in retardates than in children with normal intellectual capacity. If the brain damage that caused the retarded mental development has also caused hyperactivity and impulsivity, the combination of factors may be too much to be counteracted by even the most gentle and appropriate handling of the child. In other instances, it is understandable that the parents may have pushed the child to faster development because of their unwillingness to accept the slowness as inevitable. On reaching school age, a retarded youngster generally must first experience at least two years of failure, since in most school systems classes for children of retarded mental devlopment are not provided before

Neurosis

Clear-cut, organized neuroses are less common than behavior disorders in children. In the higher age groups, one encounters an increasing number of anxiety neuroses, obsessive-compulsive syndromes and phobias. As with the adult, the specific neurosis may be partially successful in permitting the child to deny the reality of the personality difficulties by limiting the circumstances of interaction with other persons. An example would be the hysterical youngster who has a minor fall at school and cannot walk because the school situation contains elements of intense conflict that cannot be mastered and therefore must be avoided.

Childhood Psychosis and Schizophrenic Adjustments

Childhood psychoses may be categorized as those arising from known organic causes and those in which there is no clear-cut organic etiology.

The first category includes the acute psychoses usually associated with toxicity—for example, an acute infection, or an organic brain disease of degenerative, neoplastic or traumatic nature. These psychoses are manifested in acute psychotic episodes, which have a life history determined by the nature of the underlying disease process—self-limited in an acute illness, progressive in a progressive illness. Insofar as the underlying disease is treatable, the psychosis is reversible; if the disease is progressive, as in a degenerative brain disorder, dementia is also progressive.

Among the psychoses usually classified as functional, the most frequent diagnosis is childhood schizophrenia. There has recently been a tendency to differentiate between schizophrenic adjustment and acute schizophrenic psychosis. In the several behavioral syndromes grouped under the term childhood schizophrenia, this division into psychotic and nonpsychotic would seem justified. Nevertheless, the frequency with which this formulation is at present employed suggests that it is being used as a diagnostic grab bag.

The presence of manic-depressive psychosis in young children is debatable, and the illness is generally not considered to appear earlier than adolescence. On the other hand, there have been reports of depressive reactions in infants and young children, occurring periodically and apparently closely related to traumatic situations. This has been interpreted by some psychiatrists as indicating the presence of a depressive aspect of manic-depressive psychosis before puberty.

Sociopathic Personality

If schizophrenia is the diagnostic grab bag of today, psychopathic personality was the category into which diagnostic puzzles were usually placed in the past. Particularly in the period just after World War I, the concept of the constitutional psychopath was very common. This term implied an inherent distortion in personality independent of the events occurring during the lifetime of the individual. That concept has been abandoned by most psychiatrists, and today the term sociopathic personality has largely replaced the earlier label.

The work of Lauretta Bender (1947) and William Goldfarb (1943), among others, showed that the formation of sociopathic personality in the child is often the result of environmental circumstances. It was found with macabre frequency that babies who were brought up in hospital-like situations or in frequently changing foster homes developed a constellation of behavior and personality traits which strongly resembled the behavior disturbances of the postencephalitic child. These traits included shallow interpersonal relationships, little realization of cause and effect in behavior, and, outstandingly, lack of anxiety or empathy. Such patterns were traced to the very early experiences of the infant in which he encountered constantly changing groups of people, each with their different personalities and different ways of handling him in situations that constituted an important part of his life— feeding, playing, motility, elimination. Thus, the baby presumably was trained to respond to the superficial appearance of each immediate relationship and situation. If this type of training continued over a sufficient portion of his infant life, a change to stable, consistent handling did not bring about a fundamental change in behavior.

Children with unstable, shifting early environments can be found in all socioeconomic groups. While some of these children develop sociopathic personalities, this is not true of all youngsters with such early experiences. There are also sociopathic children who come from stable homes; in these cases, the etiology of the disorder is unclear.

SELECTED REFERENCES

American Psychiatric Association: *Diagnostic and Statistical Manual of Mental Disorders.* 2nd edition. Washington, D.C., American Psychiatric Association, 1968.

Bender, L.: Psychopathic behavior disorders in children. *In* Seliger, R. V. (Ed.): *Handbook of Correctional Psychology.* New York, Philosophical Library, 1947.

Freud, A.: *Normality and Pathology in Childhood.* New York, International Universities Press, 1965.

Goldfarb, W.: Infant rearing and problem behavior. *Amer. J. Orthopsychiat.* 13:249-265, 1943.

Group for the Advancement of Psychiatry: *Psychopathological Disorders in Childhood; Theoretical Considerations and a Proposed Classification.* New York, GAP, 1966.

Kolb, L. C.: *Noyes' Modern Clinical Psychiatry.* Philadelphia, Saunders, 1968.

Shaw, C. R.: *The Psychiatric Diseases of Childhood.* New York, Appleton-Century-Crofts, 1966.

Spitzer, R. F.. and Wilson, P. T.: A guide to the American Psychiatric Association's new diagnostic nomenclature. *Amer. J. Psychiat.* 124:1619-1629, 1968.

Veith, I.: Psychiatric nosology: From Hippocrates to Kraepelin. *Amer. J. Psychiat.* 114:385-391, 1957.

World Health Organization: *International Classification of Diseases.* Geneva, WHO, 1968.

Zigler, E., and Phillips, L.: Psychiatric diagnosis: A critique. *J. Abnorm. Soc. Psychol.* 63:607-618, 1961.

9. Mental Retardation

THE UPSURGE OF INTEREST in mental retardation during the past decade has swept away many outworn dogmas in various disciplines concerned with the problem. Some healthy soul-searching has also been going on among child psychiatrists. Many of them have begun to reexamine their role in the diagnosis and rehabilitation of retarded youngsters.

Until recently, most child psychiatrists had a very limited conception of this role: that their main responsibility was to differentiate between "pseudo retardation" and "true retardation." The label "pseudo retardation" was rather indiscriminately placed on children whose intellectual deficiency was presumed to be secondary to one or another emotional disorder. Once this judgment was made, the psychiatrist proceeded to diagnose and treat the emotional disturbance, all too often without reference to the cognitive issues. On the other hand, if the child was found to have a structural incapacity for age-appropriate intellectual functioning, the psychiatrist's involvement was minimal. He considered his responsibility fulfilled when he recommended that the child be placed in a special school or institution.

This narrow approach reflected the faulty view of mental retardation as a diagnostic entity. The term is still widely used as if it referred to a unitary condition existing in a homogeneous group of persons. But the more we learn about the anatomy and biochemistry of the brain, the metabolic processes of the body as a whole, and the mechanism of heredity, the more clearly do we recognize that mental retardation is not a disease entity but an outstanding symptom of syndromes that may stem from a diversity of causes.

We have also become increasingly aware that it is essential to take into account individual differences in the temperament and behavioral style of retarded children as of all other youngsters. Closer study has exposed such global myths as that of the "quiet and contented Mongoloid." No longer is it considered sufficient to say, "He is slow intellectually; this explains his behavioral difficulties."

Psychiatrists have become more wary of such grab-bag diagnoses as "emotional block." As Leo Kanner (1956) once noted, "Somewhere along the line the term 'emotional block' was coined to indicate the masking of innate intellectual assets by psychotic or near-psychotic disturbances." Perhaps the term had some pertinence in calling attention to the fact that low IQ scores could be based on emotional factors such as anxious perfectionism or preoccupation, just as the test results could be affected by visual, auditory and neuro-orthopedic handicaps. But some professional persons, Kanner adds, have gone to the extreme of "ascribing primary emotional etiology to children who, by all standards, were, are, and will remain defective in the sense of an inherent minus." And, naturally, the mother was blamed for causing the block—another illustration of what I like to call "mal de mère." A large body of research in the past few years has reinforced our clinical awareness that the coexistence of mental subnormality and behavioral abnormality does not necessarily imply primary emotional disorder and secondary reversible retardation.

Classification

Mental retardation may be classified in terms of the degree of deficiency in intellectual functioning and also the associated clinical condition. The following classification was adopted by the American Psychiatric Association in the second edition (1968) of its *Diagnostic and Statistical Manual of Mental Disorders (DSM-II)*:

*Mental Retardation Related to IQ**

Borderline: IQ 68-85.
Mild: IQ 52-67.

---

* The IQs specified are for the Revised Stanford-Binet Tests of Intelligence, Forms L and M. Equivalent values for other tests are listed in the *Manual on Terminology and Classification in Mental Retardation* (Supplement to *American Journal of Mental Deficiency*, 2nd edition, 1961), on which DSM-II classification of mental retardation is largely based. As DSM-II emphasizes, "the intelligence quotient should not be the only criterion used in making a diagnosis of mental retardation or in evaluating its severity. It should serve only to help in making a clinical judgment of the patient's adaptive behavioral capacity. This judgment should also be based on an evaluation of the patient's developmental history and present functioning, including academic and vocational achievement, motor skills, and social and emotional maturity."

Moderate: IQ 36-51.
Severe: IQ 20-35.
Profound: IQ under 20.

Clinical Subcategories of Mental Retardation

Following infection and intoxication
Cytomegalic inclusion body disease, congenital
Rubella, congenital
Syphilis, congenital
Toxoplasmosis, congenital
Encephalopathy associated with other prenatal infections
Encephalopathy due to postnatal cerebral infection
Encephalopathy, congenital, associated with maternal toxemia
of pregnancy
Encephalopathy, congenital, associated with other maternal
intoxications
Bilirubin encephalopathy (kernicterus)
Postimmunization encephalopathy
Encephalopathy, other, due to intoxication

Following trauma or physical agent:
Encephalopathy due to prenatal injury
Encephalopathy due to mechanical injury at birth
Encephalopathy due to asphyxia at birth
Encephalopathy due to postnatal injury

With disorders of metabolism, growth, or nutrition:
Cerebral lipoidosis, infantile (Tay-Sach's disease)
Cerebral lipoidosis, late infantile (Bielschowsky's disease)
Cerebral lipoidosis, late juvenile (Kuf's disease)
Phenylketonuria
Galactosemia
Glucogenosis (Von Gierke's disease)
Hypoglycemosis

Associated with gross brain disease (postnatal):
Neurofibromatosis (von Recklinghausen's disease)
Trigeminal cerebral angiomatosis (Sturge-Weber-Dimitri's
disease)

Tuberous sclerosis
Intracranial neoplasm, other
Encephalopathy associated with diffuse sclerosis of the brain

Associated with disease and conditions due to unknown prenatal influence:

Anencephaly (including hemianencephaly)
Porencephaly, congenital
Multiple congenital anomalies of the brain
Other cerebral defects, congenital

With chromosomal abnormality:

Autosomal trisomy of Group G (Trisomy 21, Langdon-Down disease, Mongolism)
Autosomal trisomy of Group E
Autosomal trisomy of Group D
Sex chromosome anomalies
Abnormal number of chromosomes, other
Short arm deletion of chromosome 5-Group B (Cri du chat)
Short arm deletion of chromosome 18-Group E
Abnormal morphology of chromosomes, other

Associated with prematurity
Following major psychiatric disorder
With psychosocial (environmental) deprivation:

Cultural-familial mental retardation
Associated with environmental deprivation

With other (and unspecified) condition

Diagnosis

The diagnosis of retardation is based essentially on the history, clinical observation and psychologic test data.

The history may reveal that the child's development was slow from birth onward. The mothers of many children in this category have histories of difficult pregnancies or deliveries. There may be mention of neonatal stress. In many cases, however, the history may be one of normal pregnancy, delivery and neonatal period. Yet one finds that all these children have been delayed in their developmental phases, that speech in particular is slow, and that their behavior in learning situations has always been appropriate to a younger age. Physically, these children may appear normal and show no neurologic evidence of cerebral dysfunction. The vast majority of mentally retarded children fit into this category of undifferentiated or familial retardation.

A second group comprises retarded children who show neurologic signs of brain damage. This may be of a specific nature, with a special area of dysfunction, which may be neuromuscular or may involve a particular sense organ. In other cases, the symptoms may be generalized and indicate diffuse damage, with resultant disorganization of functioning that may take various forms: heightening of irritability, decrease in capacity to respond to stimuli, lessening of impulse control or decline in spontaneity.

A third category comprises children with signs of hormonal imbalance or chromosomal and metabolic abnormalities. The defect in cognition is one symptom of malfunction that modifies the brain chemistry and physiology. Psychologic tests of intelligence help identify the impaired functioning.

Another group includes children who begin life normally but show a slowing up, cessation or regression in mental development following some traumatic event, such as infection, inflammation, injury, neoplasm or degenerative neurologic disease affecting the brain. In such cases, there is a history of normal development in all areas up to the time of the brain insult. Thereafter, there is a change in the tempo of development and, eventually, a discernible pattern of retarded intellectual functioning. Clinical observation shows the child is behaving in an immature manner, and the psychologic tests confirm this finding.

These categories are useful insofar as they distinguish the kinds of problems that will confront the children as well as their parents. A child who has always been slower than average will not face the same demands as the one who has functioned normally for a number of years and only then begins to display a lag. Similarly, a child who looks normal will not necessarily have the same social difficulties as one who is palsied or has some other physical stigmata.

In making a differential diagnosis of retardation, one must be alert to certain pitfalls. A closer examination of the history may reveal that the apparently backward child is one who has always been slow to warm up to new situations. Such a child could give the impression of being retarded when he is shifted from one learning situation to another. Or a child may have a reactive behavior disorder involving his school work. He may be frightened by the newness of a classroom situation or a bad approach by the teacher. It is possible that he has been overpressured at home or overpowered by a superior sib. A full history and clinical observation may reveal adequate cognitive ability in other social situations.

The diagnosis of mental retardation must also take into account the specific nature of the child's developmental lag. For example, if he has a language lag, is this part of a general pattern of retardation or does the child handle other situations well? The diagnostician must also make sure that a child who appears retarded has intact vision and hearing. A child who is disorganized in his thinking processes is not necessarily retarded and may respond to a therapeutic program.

Children with cerebral damage may have normal IQ scores and yet be unable to handle material appropriate to their age group. They may be highly distractible and may have memory deficits or difficulty in shifting their mental set. The psychiatrist must define the handicap by estimating which learning capacities are damaged and which are intact.

For this purpose, psychologic testing is important, so long as its results are not overrated. As we all realize today, IQ test scores must be appraised with care. The tests were designed to measure a child's ability to learn in school, and there are many possible reasons why a youngster may attain a low score. I have already referred to the fact that low scores may reflect physical handicaps, specific learning disabilities and emotional factors. In addition, cultural and social biases in the tests may limit their application.

And, as Sarason (1959) pointed out, IQ scores "do not enable one to state in what ways a particular individual is different from others with an identical score, what his differential reactions are to a variety of situations, his attitudes toward himself and others." The crucial role of the psychiatrist in assessing test scores is to ask why this particular child and not others with identical IQ's behaves in the way he does, and why certain situations rather than others elicit his backward response.

Nevertheless, such psychometric testing can be of great clinical value. In some cases the test results suggest a diagnosis markedly different from what is suggested by other information available to the clinician. The person who appears dull and "looks defective" but is of average or superior IQ; the child who seems bright and glib but who fails at school and whose test results indicate that he is really a dullard despite his ready tongue; or the child who does not speak very much but whose test scores give otherwise unsuspected glimpses of latent mental capacities—these are the cases in which mental testing opens up avenues for further investigation and for remedial treatment.

Behavioral Assessment

The diagnosis of retardation is only the beginning of psychiatric exploration, not the end. Once he has identified the deficiency the psychiatrist's major responsibility still remains. This is to make a behavioral assessment of the youngster. Here his task is to determine how the fact of retardation relates to the child's over-all adaptation and development.

In considering the special problems of retarded children, the following psychiatric classification is useful:

1. Mental retardation with no behavior disorder.
2. Mental retardation with behavior symptoms that are a direct expression of organic brain damage.
3. Mental retardation with reactive behavior disorder.
4. Mental retardation with neurotic behavior disorder.
5. Mental retardation with psychosis.

While such a classification is necessarily oversimplified, it is convenient for our present purpose. It is pertinent to comment on each of these five categories.

Mental Retardation with No Behavior Disorder

Some investigators would deny that there is such a category. They assert that all retardates suffer from some specifiable psychiatric defect. For example, Thomas Webster (1963), in a study of 159 retarded children from three to six years of age, suggests that there is a primary psychopathology of mental retardation. Not one of the children, he found, was "simply retarded." Webster concludes: "The slow and incomplete unfolding of the personality is associated with partial fixations which result in an infantile or immature character structure. This particular style of ego development is accompanied by special descriptive features: a nonpsychotic autism, repetitiousness, inflexibility, passivity and simplicity in emotional life."

In my own clinical and research experiences, I have been unable to identify any emotional or behavioral characteristics that are specifically and necessarily associated with retarded children. Not all retardates have psychopathology. Moreover, not all retarded children who do have behavioral disturbances show the same symptoms. Most other workers in this field have reported varying percentages of behavior disorder among retardates, though all indicate a higher prevalence than in the general population.

What is true, of course, is that one must take into account the stresses from an environment organized primarily for the nondeviant youngster. Before his defective development has been accurately identified, the retarded child experiences a host of inappropriate demands for higher levels of performance, judgment and impulse control than lie within his capacity. Even after retardation has been established, such youngsters continue to face situations in which their inability to function in accord with age expectancy is met by displeasure and statements of disapproval. As a result of such stresses, the retarded child can be considered at risk for the development of behavioral disorders. It is the child who develops disorders that is likely to come to psychiatric attention.

Of crucial importance is the fact that behavior which is abnormal in terms of a child's chronologic age may be appropriate to his mental age. In that case, the behavioral deviance can be understood primarily in terms of the slowness of cognition. Parents are often confused about this. They may be aware that their twelve year old son is intellectually unable to assimilate formal learning, and yet may complain that he needs excessive help in dressing, whines if he is denied what he wishes, and prefers playing with five year old children in the sandbox. This youngster is at an integrated five year old level both cognitively and behaviorally. To reduce the risk that this child will develop a secondary behavior disorder, it is necessary to revise the inappropriate expectations and demands. In this respect, the technique of parent guidance is to be classified as preventive psychiatric treatment.

Mental Retardation with Behavior Disorder Due to Brain Damage

The presence of brain damage does not in itself necessarily mean that there will be disordered behavior. Some youngsters with clinically demonstrable brain damage, as evidenced by the various types of congenital cerebral palsy, may be behaviorally well adjusted. Others may show a wide range of behaviors that are direct symptoms of faulty cerebral functioning. Similarly, retarded children with brain damage may exhibit such diverse symptoms of organic dysfunction as hypermobility or hypomotility, brevity or excessive length of attention span, high distractibility or imperviousness to environmental stimuli, hyperirritability or hypoirritability, lability of mood or monotonous sameness, excessive dependence on people or inappropriate independence. Obsessive thoughts and compulsive behaviors are also to be seen in such children, as manifested in repetitive questions, stereotyped gestures or mechanically rhythmic body movements.

Some of these symptoms can be modified by psychopharmacologic agents. It may be possible, for example, to decrease activity, increase attention span, lessen emotional lability and ameliorate depression through a drug regimen. In large part, however, the treatment of organically determined symptoms involves milieu therapy; that is, organizing a way of life with appropriately modified expectations that take into account the child's vulnerabilities as well as his abilities. Thus, the child with short attention span should be presented with new demands only in brief teaching episodes; the hyperirritable child must be shielded from intense scolding; the hypoactive child should be given intense stimulation.

Mental Retardation with Reactive Disorder

When the retarded child enters the world of his peers, the social meaning of his slowness begins to take form. Even if he escapes being made fun of in his preschool years, his inability to keep up in the area of formal learning will make him a target for jeers in the classroom. The child's parents, reluctant to accept his handicap, may handle him inappropriately. Misunderstanding his capacity, embarrassed about community reaction, they may keep the child from joining groups made up of his intellectual peers.

It is not surprising that intellectually handicapped children tend to build up a host of defensive behavior patterns. Retarded children, like the rest of us, may be happy or sad, aggressive or docile, adventurous or timid. But an unhealthy interaction between child and environment can distort feelings, turning happiness into clowning, sadness into depression. Either docility or aggression may become a way of life, and timidity may be converted to fear and anxiety.

Unfortunately, we do not have nearly enough systematic information on the factors responsible for the development of behavioral disturbances in mentally retarded children. A great deal has been written on the influence of emotional factors on intellectual functioning, but very little on the effect that mental retardation may have upon psychologic functioning and personality development. The influence of parents on the retarded child's emotional life has been extensively described, but one-sidedly in terms of acceptance versus rejection of the child and the effect of guilt and anxiety feelings.

That parental love and acceptance are essential for the healthy psychologic development of any child is well established. But it is a dangerous simplification to jump to the conclusion that parental love can always overcome the stressful effects of all difficulties confronting the child. Parents of retarded children must cope with special demands of time, energy, emotional living, ingenuity in planning and money. To offer parents the illusory hope that these stresses will disappear with love and acceptance can lead only to cruel disappointment, confusion, and self-blame.

In planning a therapeutic program for retarded children with reactive behavior disorders, one must identify the specific functioning of the child that has led to and exacerbated the negative interaction of child and environment. One must define the aspects of behavioral organization that bear on the child's capacity to respond to environmental demands.

Few attempts have been made to do this in a systematic way. One such attempt was a six year research project, funded by the National Institute of Mental Health, in which the author was the principal investigator. We studied a sample of fifty-two retarded children living at home with their middle-class intact families. The chronologic ages of the children ranged from five and a half to eleven and a half years; their IQ scores from 50 to 75; and their mental ages from four to six years. All the children attended special classes in public and private schools. The nature of the sample was advantageous for the purpose of identifying features of behavioral organization that bear a relationship to mental abnormality as such. It was possible to exclude a number of variables that could contaminate the behavioral findings. Such possibly contaminating variables include: (a) environmental stress produced by marginal economic status or family disorganization; (b) past failure to diagnose the existence of retardation, resulting in a history of unrealistic demands and expectations; (c) institutionalization, which may in itself affect behavioral development; and (d) the existence of significant degrees of motor handicap or physical stigmata, which may create special stresses in attempts at environmental mastery and social functioning.

Thirty-one children were diagnosed as having a behavior problem. Of these, nine had behavior problems that were direct symptoms of cerebral dysfunction, nineteen had reactive behavior disorders, two had neurotic behavior disorders and one was psychotic.

One striking finding was the frequency with which professional workers consulted by the family had avoided the diagnosis of mental retardation. This phenomenon became evident as we established contact with special schools, recreational facilities and organizations for mentally retarded children, and as we received reports from psychiatrists, psychologists, social workers and educators. Parents had often been told that the child's basic problem was one of emotional disturbance and that the mental retardation was a secondary phenomenon; i.e., our old friend "pseudo retardation." In general, the professional literature deals with the problem of parents who refuse to accept the diagnosis of retardation in their child. Very little attention, however, is given to the problem of professional workers who show this bias in favor of a diagnosis of emotional disturbance.

We also found to our surprise that there is a widespread lack of understanding that the *degree* of intellectual retardation is a significant factor in determining the child's adaptive capacities and potential for coping with the demands of his environment. This would appear to be self-evident, but we noted many instances in which psychiatrists and social workers gave guidance and treatment without obtaining a reliable psychometric evaluation.

To determine the children's levels of functioning in self-care, socialization, play, etc., we found it necessary to distinguish between the level of habitual functioning and the child's actual capacity. This differentiation is not made in the performance scales currently in use, such as the Vineland Social Maturity Scale. Our data indicate that this distinction is an important one. For example, a child was reported by the parent to be able to dress himself completely. However, this was not a routine accomplishment but possible only under optimum conditions at home. At school, faced with many distractions and noise, the child required help. Overestimation of a youngster's abilities, by confusing his highest level of functioning with his routine level, may lead to excessive expectations and demands. On the other hand, exclusive consideration of the child's routine abilities may lead to an underestimation of his capacities and the setting of inadequate goals.

As noted in earlier chapters, one of the significant factors entering into any child-environment interactional process is the attribute of temperament. The behavioral records in the study of fifty-two children showed that these youngsters, too, could be characterized in terms of their style of reaction to varied situations of day-to-day living. Qualitative analysis of the data in the children with behavioral disturbances indicates quite clearly that temperamental factors play a significant role in the development of such disturbances in interaction with environmental stresses and, in some cases, the special behavioral consequences of brain damage.

To illustrate, one child had frequent tantrums that expressed a characteristically negative response to the new and unfamiliar. The parents dealt with this problem by shielding her from new experiences. She had fewer tantrums, but the lack of new stimuli and learning experiences resulted in a level of functioning below her potential capacity. The parents were advised to expose her to selectively graded new situations by stages and gently, and to expect tantrums the first few times. With this appropriate management, the child was given the optimally structured learning atmosphere for her temperament and intellectual level.

Another child, on the other hand, adapted quickly to new situations and functioned easily with simple routine tasks. He was also an extremely persistent child, and this, in combination with his retarded level of learning, resulted in his sticking to a difficult task in a perseverative, repetitive fashion without mastery. As a consequence, his IQ level gradually decreased from a score of 75 at six years to one of 57 at age nine years, six months, and he also developed a number of perseverative behavior patterns. Treatment involved guiding his parents and teachers to divide every new task into small sequential segments, each of which he could master in turn and then pass on to the next segment.

It should be noted that in some cases diminished intellectual function may be a consequence of a reactive behavior disorder. For example, a child may react directly to an abrupt shift in environmental circumstances by developing a defensive maneuver of intellectual immobility. Thus, one Negro child from the South having his first classroom contact with a white teacher in the North, was frightened into temporary paralysis of his learning ability. Another youngster, who was very shy, was shocked into protective immobility by a shouting teacher, only to return to good functioning with a soft-spoken teacher.

Mental Retardation with Neurotic Behavior Disorder

This combination may occur in two sequences: (a) the mentally retarded child who develops a neurotic pattern of behavior; and (b) the youngster who develops neurotic behavior patterns which lead to lowered intellectual functioning.

While the reactive behavior disorders can be modified by altering the environmental organization, neurotic behavior disorders show more firmly fixed patterns and may not be so amenable to change. Neurotic manifestations may reflect anxieties or defenses against anxiety. The child may be fearful in all new situations or in specific types of situations. He may have phobic reactions or rigid attitudes inappropriate to the intentions or actions of those around him.

In all cases, however, one must guard against misinterpreting acts that are appropriate to a given mental age as neurotic behavior in a retarded child. These acts may appear to reflect neurotic attitudes only because they are incongruous with a youngster's actual age and physical appearance.

For the mentally retarded child who is indeed neurotic, direct psychotherapy may be advisable. Although psychotherapy is not commonly recommended for mentally retarded children, I can report a measure of success with this approach. To be sure, the techniques of psychotherapy with normal children require modification for effective application to retarded youngsters. The goals of such treatment must be individualized, with full recognition that the child will continue to function on a retarded level. It is important that we do not give false hopes to the parents.

However, in many cases, the anxiety and fears of retarded children can be alleviated, no matter how limited the child's intelligence, so that he can be included in some approximation of normal family life. In general, the child's intellectual level will determine whether it is possible to reach him in conceptual terms, or whether relationship therapy or some form of conditioning will be more effective.

Strong, rigid, neurotic defenses prevent the optimal use of a nonretarded child's intellectual capacity. If such inhibition of intellectual functioning is severe, the child may operate on a level of mental retardation. The average child is keenly interested in the world around him and has spent his preschool life in very active learning experiences. But if his experience in the course of eager exploration has created the concept that the world is a dangerous place, he may feel that safety lies in sticking to the tried and proved, an attitude that interferes with the acquisition of knowledge and gives the impression of incapacity to learn. Similarly, a child who has found that mistakes are not to be tolerated may be so afraid to hazard a guess that he will not reach out for new experiences. An extreme degree of competitiveness or fear of authority figures may interfere with the learning process. A sense of inferiority engendered by rivalry with a sibling who is alert, bright and quick may cause a youngster to take for himself the role of the stupid one. These and a host of other neurotic mechanisms may be the cause of retarded function in a child of normal or better than normal capacity. In such cases, adequate treatment of the neurotic difficulty may result in more successful use of the intellectual potential. By the same token, a retarded child may be functioning below his capacity as a result of neurotic defenses, and successful treatment would enable him to function at a higher though still retarded level.

Mental Retardation with Psychosis

In children in whom both subnormal intellectual functioning and childhood psychosis are present, the decision as to which is to be considered primary and which secondary is often purely semantic and may not determine the treatment plans or goals. For the youngster with an autistic type of disorder, one may postulate that the achievement of increased awareness of the people and activities around him would result in better cognitive functioning. Planned stimuli in this direction would indeed be appropriate treatment. This can be attempted through enrollment of the child in a recreation group, specified parental interaction, speech, music or dance therapy, or direct psychotherapy. How much any of these programs will accomplish, however, may depend on the severity and irreversibility of the syndrome, factors about which our knowledge is still limited.

Other children with both psychosis and subnormal cognitive functioning may require treatment designed to give them maximum superimposition of structure with a view to limiting their freely wandering flights of thought and activity.

In recent years, much attention has been focused on childhood schizophrenia as a cause of retardation. We have long lists of youngsters whose condition is diagnosed as "childhood schizophrenia." The belief that schizophrenia is relatively treatable is so firmly held by many parents, as well as some professional groups, that the psychiatrist is often pressured into replacing a diagnosis of mental retardation by one of childhood schizophrenia. Inattention and unresponsiveness to the environment is called "mutism," peculiarities of speech and motility are dubbed "bizarre," an occasional response of obvious relevance and logic is seen as a "flash of normal intelligence," and a diagnosis of "schizophrenia" is born which is invoked almost as a magic talisman to ward off the evil of permanent disability.

It is certainly true that a proportion of the population in institutions for the mentally retarded are basically schizophrenic. Since learning requires communication of knowledge from one person to another, a severe interference with interpersonal communication will decrease one's ability to learn. The highest degree of this difficulty is found in autistic youngsters.

But it is sometimes difficult to make a differential diagnosis. A retarded child may have a vacant look in his eyes that may make him appear to be autistic. Yet his failure to respond does not necessarily mean autism in the sense that he is self-preoccupied. It may merely mean that his degree of retardation is such that he does not have the capacity to react to certain external stimuli. Such terms as autism, echolalia and echopraxia have become so firmly associated with childhood schizophrenia as to impede careful diagnostic evaluation. In many instances, once a child has been described as exhibiting echolalia, the diagnosis of schizophrenia has to all intents and purposes been made. The fact that echolalia is a normal way of learning speech and that it is therefore not unexpected in a retardate who is mastering speech may easily be forgotten in the reliance on the presumed pathognomonic symptom.

In our study of fifty-two retarded children, we observed that their language functioning was more retarded than their nonverbal behavior. Also notable in our sample was the degree to which speech was repetitive, perseverative and stereotyped, even though other aspects of their behavior were organized and affectively responsive. Since there is a penchant for using these speech characteristics as indices to diagnose emotional disturbance and mutism, it is important to note their presence in psychiatrically normal but mentally retarded children. If perseverative and stereotyped verbal patterns are automatically assumed to be signs of emotional disorder or disorganization of thought process, there is a great danger that psychiatric treatment will be arranged for a child who really needs an effective educational and management program.

While much perseverative speech is to be found in both retarded and autistic children, there are essential differences in the kind of repetition as well as in the behavioral context. Autistic repetition appears to have no aim beyond the activity itself and resembles the preintentional behavior patterns which occur in the early infancy of normal children, whereas the delayed echolalia of retarded children does have some relevance and is less purely a matter of lifting phrases out of context and repeating them. Schizophrenic children show affective withdrawal and deficient socialization, but retarded children try to convey ideas, are competent in the simple tasks of daily living and display appropriate affectivity.

A grossly retarded child may appear bizarre. The incongruity between physical appearance and aimless running about or repetitive actions can be very striking. But if the observed behavior of a retarded child would seem appropriate in a child of a younger chronologic age, then it cannot accurately be called bizarre. Nor does the existence of single repetitive pattern mean that the child is autistic. The same child may help his mother put the groceries away and may also participate in all sorts of social acts. This is not a schizophrenic child, but a retarded youngster with special habit patterns.

It must also be remembered that childhood schizophrenia is itself not a single disease, and that its treatability varies. Even if a child is correctly transferred from the retardate to the schizophrenic group, the prognosis may not be altered. In any case, the issue is not whether the diagnosis makes the prognosis more helpful, but whether the diagnosis is correct. If a retarded child is treated for schizophrenia, appropriate plans for management and vocational guidance may be unnecessarily postponed.

The diagnosis of retardation and the degree of severity should be conveyed to parents without camouflage. The prevention and treatment of emotional problems of the retarded child requires an orientation toward using the parent as a colleague.

To begin with, it is pertinent to make a detailed inventory of the data available for each child including: (1) IQ level and any special characteristics of perceptual and cognitive functioning revealed by the psychometric testing; (2) the level of functioning in various activities of daily living—both the maximum and the habitual level; (3) temperamental characteristics; (4) learning pattern, including the manner in which the child himself identifies errors and seeks to correct them, as well as his response to correction by others; (5) patterns of parental practices and techniques of dealing with the child's problems; (6) special intrafamilial or extrafamilial environmental stresses; and (7) relevant features of medical, neurologic and psychiatric examinations.

The child's problems can be evaluated in terms of the interrelationship and interactions of these factors. On the basis of this analysis, the discussion with the parents focuses on making them aware of the demands and expectations that are easy, difficult or impossible for the child to master. A program of activity is then laid out with the goal of increasing the child's ability to master difficult demands and to cope with stress through an alteration in parental functioning. The extent of this program is of course contingent on an estimate of the parents' capacities to follow concrete directions for change in their handling and on their ability to maintain a new approach consistently. While generalizations regarding "acceptance" of the retarded child may be useful, they are of limited value. A program of altered parental function, spelled out concretely and based on an analysis of the individual child-environment interaction, offers useful possibilities for helping the retarded child cope most constructively with the special stresses and demands of his life.

SELECTED REFERENCES

American Psychiatric Association: *Diagnostic and Statistical Manual of Mental Disorders.* 2nd Edition. Washington, D.C., American Psychiatric Association, 1968.

Chess, S.: Psychiatric treatment of the mentally retarded child with behavior problems. *Amer. J. Orthopsychiat.* 32:863-869, 1962.

Clarke, A. M., and Clarke, A. D. B. (Eds.): *Mental Deficiency: The Changing Outlook.* New York, The Free Press, 1965.

Ellis, N. R. (Ed.): *Handbook of Mental Deficiency.* New York, McGraw-Hill, 1963.

Heber, R.: *A Manual on Terminology and Classification in Mental Retardation.* Washington, American Association on Mental Deficiency, 1961.

Hermelin, B. F., and O'Connor, N.: *Speech and Thought in Severe Subnormality.* Oxford, Pergamon Press, 1963.

Hilliard, L. T., and Kirman, B. H.: *Mental Deficiency.* London, Churchill, 1965.

Kanner, L.: *A Miniature Textbook of Feeblemindedness.* Child Care Monographs, No. 1. New York, Child Care Publications, 1949.

Kanner, L.: The "emotional block." *Amer. J. Psychiat.* 113:181-182, 1956.

Penrose, L. S.: *The Biology of Mental Defect.* New York, Grune & Stratton, 1962.

Sarason, S. B.: *Psychological Problems in Mental Deficiency.* New York, Harper, 1959.

Tredgold, R. F., and Soddy, K.: *A Textbook of Mental Deficiency.* London, Balliere, Tindall & Cox, 1963.

Webster, T.: Problems of emotional development in young retarded children. *Amer. J. Psychiat.* 120:37-43, 1963.

Zigler, E.: Familial mental retardation: a continuing dilemma. *Science* 155:292-298, 1967.

10. Behavioral Disorders Due to Cerebral Dysfunction

ALTHOUGH CHILDREN with cerebral dysfunction often present behavior problems requiring special diagnosis and treatment, it should not be assumed that brain disease or injury necessarily leads to behavioral aberrations. On the contrary, many brain-damaged children are able to make a healthy adjustment to their circumstances, and the only functional distortions may be in motor activity.

The causal relationship between cerebral dysfunction and behavior disorder is more readily recognized in some organic disturbances than in others. Extensive injury may be directly linked to grossly aberrant manifestations in behavioral, perceptual, motor or cognitive areas. In other instances, a behavioral disturbance may not be caused by the lesion itself, but may be reactive to the limitations or distortions of functioning that it produces. Often the total behavioral problem combines the direct behavioral symptoms of brain damage and the defensive set of actions against the circumstances produced by the structural difficulty. The severity of these disturbances varies considerably.

In many cases, the behavioral disturbance comes to notice first. It is then the child psychiatrist's responsibility to identify the fact of an organic etiology and arrange for investigations to determine the nature and degree of neurologic damage. On the other hand, children with an already known neurologic deficit may develop problems of behavior. The psychiatrist must then differentiate between the structural difficulty and the social problems arising from organic limitations or distortions of capacity.

Sometimes this distinction is easy to make. When a child has a degenerative disease of the brain, his loss of interest in his surroundings and his lowered intellectual functioning are readily understood as direct symptoms of the organic changes. In the epileptic child, irritability in personality makeup may be a direct result of brain irritation. When brain tissue is destroyed by an injury or a tumor, functioning formerly controlled by the affected portion of the brain is disrupted.

A brain lesion, however, does not necessarily lead to behavioral disturbances. Even when hard neurologic signs are present, one cannot automatically conclude that a specific behavioral disorder will follow in the wake of damage. On the other hand, one must be aware that behavioral consequences of neurologic damage may be delayed. For example, a child who has had encephalitis may recover without any noticeable organic sequelae, yet he may later show behavioral symptoms such as great impulsiveness, shortened attention span, proneness to distraction, hyperactivity, slow reactivity, lethargy or shallowness of mood. These or other symptoms may appear after recovery from a severe burn in which toxicity has been demonstrated by high fever and delirium. They may also occur after a hematoma or brain laceration, or after carbon monoxide or lead poisoning. The symptoms are sometimes found in cases in which there is only a vague possibility that there was anoxia at birth. Epidemiologic studies indicate that behavior problems may be related to prenatal and perinatal complications that have not resulted in clear-cut organic damage.

Observations of children who had suffered known cerebral insults led to the description of the "hyperkinetic" syndrome. Strauss and Werner (1941) were the first to delineate the behavioral sequelae of minimal central nervous system damage in children. The investigators included as "brain-damaged" those youngsters who were hyperactive, emotionally labile, perceptually disordered, impulsive and distractible. As Eisenberg (1964) notes, these findings led to an unfortunate syllogism: "Children with known brain damage exhibit, or may exhibit, such and such behavior; the patient under study displays similar behavior; ergo, he is brain damaged." There has been a persistent tendency to refer to all minimally brain-damaged children as a unitary group characterized as hyperkinetic and to diagnose any hyperkinetic child as brain-damaged, often through circular reasoning.

The common assumption of a "hyperkinetic" syndrome has recently come under scrutiny. Various workers (Birch, 1964; Eisenberg, 1964) now emphasize the paucity of evidence that children who exhibit the Straussian pattern do, in fact, have brain damage. Many children with organic damage that has been verified through neurologic or anatomic examination do not exhibit the patterns of behavior presumably characteristic of this defect. While hyperkinesis frequently comes to clinical notice, it is neither synonymous with nor pathognomonic for brain damage. The syndromes displayed by children with cerebral dysfunction are extremely varied.

A number of investigators have disputed the view, once widely accepted, that all brain lesions, wherever localized, are followed by a similar kind of disordered behavior. Just as the organic damage varies with the size, locus and type of lesion, so, too, may the behavioral syndromes. Behavioral indices as criteria for brain damage are insufficient, since not all brain-damaged children show signs of behavior impairment. To describe hyperkinesis as the major response to brain damage is an oversimplification.

The recognition of diversity is crucial for avoiding two major pitfalls. First, if a child with classic signs of hyperkinesis is automatically diagnosed as brain-damaged, the clinician may fail to perform a detailed evaluation of the youngster's functioning. He may overlook the need to examine the specific ways in which the child's symptoms are manifested: Are they attentional or perceptual? Is the youngster unable to carry in his mind more than a certain number of directions at a time? Is he impulsive? All aspects of the child's functioning must be considered in formulating an appropriate therapeutic program. In some cases, the hyperactive child will be brain-damaged, and this evaluation will color whatever therapy is recommended. In other children, however, the "symptoms" of cerebral dysfunction may represent a nonpathologic extension of temperamental characteristics. The treatment of these children will be based on a faulty diagnosis if the judgment of brain damage is left standing.

The second pitfall in equating hyperkinesis with brain damage is that the investigator may fail to pursue a full differential diagnosis in the case of a nonhyperkinetic child who "doesn't act like a brain-damaged youngster." The possibility of brain dysfunction should not be ruled out merely because a behaviorally disturbed child fails to show the classic signs of hyperkinesis.

The pertinence of these warnings is suggested by a review of 1,307 patients seen in the author's consultation practice. The review had a twofold aim: (1) to see how many of the children had neurologic damage (ascertained through history of some insult, positive neurologic findings, X-ray or EEG abnormalities); and (2) to survey the behavioral manifestations of these children. Eighty-nine (6.8 per cent) of the children were found to have brain damage. The presenting problems covered a wide range. Forty children were said to be hyperactive and fifty-nine showed aggressive behavior, a category that is often congruent with hyperactivity. (These and the following figures are overlapping, as several children showed more than one symptom.) Nonhyperactive, nonaggressive children also were well represented. Fifteen youngsters were described as dependent, eighteen as withdrawn, twenty-four were said to have no friends, and two were beaten up by other children.

Abnormalities and delays in development also represented a high proportion of the presenting problems. Forty-four children had past or present speech delays or disturbances, fifty had past or present motoric delays or disturbances, and fourteen showed other abnormalities of development sufficiently troublesome to the parents to warrant their seeking psychiatric consultation. Of the total group of children, fifty-seven had some representation of anxieties, fears, phobias, obsessions, compulsions or other neurotic symptoms. Sixty children had academic difficulties.

These findings must be considered in light of the general description of the brain-damaged child as one who has a short attention span and is hyperactive, impulsive and emotionally labile. Obviously, the practicing psychiatrist does not see a wide sample of all children with neurologic damage, but only those who are having or are giving trouble. As a result, one would anticipate that among those youngsters who are brought to psychiatric attention, there would be a high preponderance of these so-called "nuisance" children who are likely to find themselves in difficulty in structured situations that require impulse control, attention span, direction-following and the ability to sit still. The school-age child, especially, would be expected to have a high proportion of such presenting problems. It is noteworthy, therefore, that although the hyperkinetic syndrome did occur in some children as a consequence of central nervous system damage, it by no means constituted the invariable result of such damage. The behavioral sequelae were diverse.

Similarly, in a review of hospitalized children for whom organic factors appeared important to their clinical state, Pond (1961) reports that the "symptoms are extraordinarily varied, and it is clear at once that the classical syndrome of the brain-damaged child does not cover more than a few of the children seen." In view of the wide range of behavioral patterns that a brain-damaged child may display, how can one make a valid rather than presumptive diagnosis of organicity? As Clements (1966) has stated, "The 'sign' approach can serve only as a guideline for the purpose of identification and diagnosis." Much will depend on the performance of a rigorous and comprehensive diagnostic evaluation that includes both medical and behavioral assessments.

One must guard against making a one-to-one relationship between the behavioral and cerebral symptoms. The behavioral symptoms depend partly on the area of the brain involved, partly on the extent and nature of the lesion, and partly on the child's personality before the onset of illness. In addition, the child-environment interaction plays a role. The major problem is to distinguish between psychologic symptoms resulting directly from brain injury and those that are secondary reactions.

In assessing behavioral symptoms, consideration should be given to the functional impairment resulting from extensive destruction of brain tissue, regardless of the localization of the loss. The child with extensive brain damage may be unable to accomplish complex tasks or several tasks simultaneously, although he can handle tasks presented singly. The explanation of this phenomenon advanced by Eisenberg (1957) is that if a large number of the nerve pathways employed in common by impulses originating from many different points are destroyed as a result of mass tissue loss, messages cannot always be transmitted. The central nervous system may be thought of as a complex of transient electrical fields whose reciprocal interrelation is necessary for normal functioning. Any distortion in the network of the cortex is likely to alter the individual's social adaptability.

Cerebral dysfunction may have various manifestations. Intellectual functioning may be impaired, or there may be defects in muscular functioning, flaccid or spastic paralysis, tremors, athetosis in the muscles of locomotion, of speech, or of the eyes. There are innumerable combinations of malfunctioning.

The secondary symptoms of avoidance, clowning, negativism, and withdrawal may extend the brain-damaged child's handicap beyond the area of the primary defect. For example, a child who has difficulty in concentration or coordination may assume a passive, dependent role, letting others do his thinking and acting. He is likely to feel that he cannot carry out tasks or take care of himself. A child with uncontrollable muscular impulses that make writing difficult may refuse to use the special pencil devised to minimize his difficulty, and he may have a temper tantrum whenever attention is focused on his weakness. Brain-damaged children who continually experience partial failure because of their handicap may tend to freeze into silence, or they may show overt symptoms of anxiety. Such symptoms may be secondary to the basic handicap; they may also be direct expressions of the brain dysfunction.

The problem of distinguishing the primary from the secondary symptoms is compounded in children with minimal cerebral dysfunction. These children are usually of near average, average or even above average intelligence and have various behavioral or learning disabilities, ranging from mild to severe, associated with central nervous system deviations. Their organic symptoms are minor or mild and can be grouped in five major categories: (1) impairment of fine movement or coordination; (2) electroencephalographic abnormalities; (3) deviations in attention, activity level or affect; (4) perceptual, intellectual and memory deficits; and (5) nonperipheral sensory impairments. Their behavioral symptoms can be grouped into the following major categories: hyperactivity, perceptual-motor impairments, emotional lability, general coordination deficits, disorders of attention (distractibility, perseveration), impulsivity, disorders of memory and thinking, specific learning disabilities, disorders of speech and hearing, equivocal neurologic signs.

One cannot look for a single indication of organicity. Only a complete evaluation of the child will reveal any causative factors of disease or injury that can be prevented or ameliorated. Only such an evaluation makes it possible to define the child's physical or intellectual limitations and thus to organize a remedial program.

The fact that the diagnosis of cerebral dysfunction may be judgmental rather than definitive in many cases should not blur the importance of obtaining comprehensive histories. These should include complete medical, developmental and family records; general and neurologic physical examinations; special sensory and laboratory tests, including X-rays and electroencephalographs; psychologic testing; and a thorough behavioral assessment. Separate findings may not in themselves be conclusive. Past damage cannot in itself be claimed as the cause of subsequent symptoms; verbal-performance discrepancies are found in non-brain-damaged children and brain-damaged children do not always have them; perceptual tests are not always adequate. But a combination of several suspicious findings does indicate that organicity must be considered in the diagnostic evaluation and treatment plan.

In cases with no clear-cut organic history or neurologic findings, the psychologic tests—particularly the Bender Gestalt Test for visual-motor coordination and the Goldstein-Scheerer Tests of abstract and concrete behavior—may give the best diagnostic clues. Disturbances in hand and eye coordination, poor perception of form, difficulty in concentration and other symptoms of organic brain disturbance may show up in bold relief in the testing situation. But it must be kept in mind that many of these findings are also symptomatic of anxiety. If there is no confirmatory evidence of brain damage, a differential diagnosis may be extremely difficult.

Yet it is of prime importance to differentiate between neurotic anxiety and behavior disturbance resulting from brain damage, since the two disorders call for quite different treatment. The child whose anxiety is caused by vague awareness that his functioning is impaired will benefit—and his anxiety may be relieved—by treatment appropriate for a brain-damaged child. But if anxiety is the cause rather than the effect of deviations in functioning, treatment must focus on resolving the conflicts at the root of the anxiety.

As part of the New York Longitudinal Study, my colleagues and I were able to follow the developmental course of three brain-damaged children from early infancy into the school years. The data available on each child included behavioral characteristics, patterns of parental performance, neurologic and psychiatric manifestations, and psychometric status. This study sought to identify factors in development contributing to the different types of behavioral influences as opposed to those on a more physiologic level. Each of the children was representative of a different type of developmental course that may attend neurologic damage acquired in early life. It was concluded that in every instance the child's temperamental organization was useful as a predictor of the developmental course, and that the temperament-environment interaction was a crucial factor in the behavioral outcomes.

Therapeutic Approaches

Several decades ago, the brain-damaged child was treated only for the organic components of his illness, generally by a pediatrician or neurologist. No attempt was made to deal with the behavioral components, since these were considered unalterable. Today, child psychiatrists are more optimistic about the possibility of alleviating the behavioral difficulties. This change of attitude has resulted partly from better understanding of the course of brain disease, but chiefly from the development of new treatment techniques.

In some diseases of the brain, the organic component offers no possibility of improvement through medical treatment, but the behavioral factor remains available for treatment and should not be ignored. In other diseases, the organic component responds completely or partially to medical measures, but the disease leaves in its wake a prominent behavior disorder that becomes the most pressing complaint. In either event, the prognosis may range from very poor to very good, and such children are entitled to the best available therapeutic efforts.

We are indebted to Lauretta Bender (1956) for some of our optimistic concepts about the treatability of brain-damaged children and to Kurt Goldstein (1954) for detailed studies of rehabilitation procedures. Successful work is based on the premise that hyperactivity which cannot be eliminated can at least be channeled. The child who has been unable to function in normal society because of his impulsiveness can make a better adjustment if both he and those around him learn to recognize incipient signs of uncontrollable restlessness and if a constructive outlet for his impulses is provided. When this procedure is followed, secondary symptomatology such as negativism or hostility can be kept to a minimum.

The aim of psychiatric treatment for the child with cerebral dysfunction is to help him take his place in normal society insofar as his handicap permits. If this cannot be attained and the young patient cannot lead a normal existence, special facilities must be utilized so that he can grow up in an environment tailored to his needs. Even in such an environment, relationships with normal children should be fostered to the extent possible. Ideally, the child should attend the community school and take part in neighborhood recreational activities.

Attempts to provide a normal environment and normal contacts for brain-injured children often fail because of social attitudes. Chief among the deterrent factors is the litigation-consciousness of our present society. Many educational and recreational institutions hesitate to accept a child who is known to have a convulsive disorder lest an injury to him expose them to a lawsuit. Similarly, a hyperactive and impulsive child is often unwelcome in supervised group activities of normal children because of the fear that he may accidentally injure another child. These and many other factors over and above the brain-damaged child's own capacities must be taken into account in attempts to provide a normal environment.

The most prominent manifestations of disturbance in the organically damaged child at the time of referral may be the mechanisms of avoidance, clowning, negativism and withdrawal. In all likelihood, such a youngster's self-esteem is low, and he tends to use whatever psychologic defenses he can muster. Hence, the initial treatment sessions generally aim to give him a feeling that he is worthwhile and that he has some positive attributes. This objective must be at least partly achieved before the child can confront his disability and attempt to minimize its social consequences.

Treatment efforts are directed toward helping the child gain a clear concept of the nature and degree of his handicap in terms of his chronologic or mental age, and an understanding of his own capacity—what he himself can handle and what warrants a request for aid. He should be able to distinguish between those situations in which he can compete with his peers on an equal basis, those in which he can participate only in a modified way, and those in which he must perforce be an onlooker. He should be helped to channel his uncontrollable functions in order to minimize their negative social consequences.

Other procedures than psychotherapy may be indicated in the treatment of children with cerebral dysfunction. Drug treatment is particularly worth mentioning. Many reports have indicated that the amphetamines are effective in the treatment of hyperactivity. By some paradoxic action, they appear to decrease the activity level and increase the attention span of these children. Similarly, pharmacologic agents may be used to control the seizures of epileptic children. Naturally, one must justify their use by determining how well they control the convulsive disorder and what their side effects are.

The most favorable results in treating brain-damaged children are often obtained by the combined use of medication, psychotherapy and parent guidance. Whether carried out formally or informally, parent guidance is of particular importance. One of the first steps is to explain the organic difficulties and their functional significance in terms that will give the parents an awareness of what may realistically be expected of the child. The parents must be told that while the impairment is defined in terms of the child's age level at the time of consultation, the functional difficulties will change as he goes through successive stages of maturation and is confronted with varying demands. Thus, a defect has to be interpreted in terms of both its present and future implications. The professional offering guidance must identify the indications of changing capacity in the child and help the parents to modify their methods of handling in response to the change.

The treatment program emphasizes the fullest development of the child's positive characteristics in order to enhance his chances for optimum adaptation. One must avoid applying a general formula to all children who display cerebral dysfunction and attendant behavioral manifestations. Just as there is no unitary brain-damage syndrome, so, too, there is no single cure for all children in all circumstances. Each child must be dealt with in terms of his own temperament and his own particular defect. Each set of parents must be guided in terms of their personalities and the specific characteristics of the child. It will not do to offer a blanket prescription of nonpermissiveness, as many authors have done. Only when the brain-injured child is recognized as an individual reactive being will there be a reasonable chance of ameliorating the secondary effects of his cerebral dysfunction and helping him to function healthily and adaptively.

SELECTED REFERENCES

Bender, L.: *Psychopathology of Children with Organic Brain Disorders.* Springfield, Ill., Charles C Thomas, 1956.

Birch, H. G. (Ed.): *Brain Damage in Children.* Baltimore, Williams & Wilkins, 1964.

Bortner, M. (Ed.): *Evaluation and Education of Children with Brain Damage.* Springfield, Ill., Charles C Thomas, 1968.

Clements, S. D.: *Minimal Brain Dysfunction in Children.* Washington, Department of Health, Education and Welfare, Public Health Service Publication No. 1415, 1966.

Eisenberg, L.: Psychiatric implications of brain damage in children. *Psychiat. Quart.* 31:75, 1957.

Eisenberg, L.: Behavioral manifestations of cerebral damage in childhood. *In* Birch, H. G. (Ed.): *Brain Damage in Children,* Baltimore, Williams & Wilkins, 1964.

Goldstein, K.: The brain-injured child. *In* Michal-Smith, H. (Ed.): *Pediatric Problems in Clinical Practice.* New York, Grune & Stratton, 1954.

Pasamanick, B., and Knobloch, H.: Epidemiologic studies on the complications of pregnancy and the birth process. *In* Caplan, G. (Ed.): *Prevention of Mental Disorders in Children.* New York, Basic Books, 1961.

Pond, D. A.: Psychiatric aspects of epileptic and brain-damaged children. *Brit. Med. J.* 5265:1454, 1961.

Strauss, A. A., and Kephart, N. C.: *Psychopathology and Education of the Brain Injured Child.* Vol. 2., *Progress in Theory and Clinic.* New York, Grune & Stratton, 1955.

Strauss, A. A., and Lehtinen, L.: *Psychopathology and Education of the Brain Injured Child,* Vol. I. New York, Grune & Stratton, 1950.

Strauss, A. A., and Werner, H.: The mental organization of the brain-injured mentally defective child. *Amer. J. Psychiat.* 97:1194, 1941.

11. Behavior and Character Disorders, Neuroses, and Associated Symptoms

IN BROAD PERSPECTIVE, the behavior disorders of children may be viewed as a progression of increasing complexity. At one end of the continuum is the basically normal child who is neither brain-damaged, mentally retarded nor schizophrenic, but who does have a characteristic pattern of behavior that is causing management problems. At the other end is a disturbed child with a sociopathic character disorder. In between are children with reactive behavior disorders of varying severity, neurotic behavior disorders, neuroses, neurotic character disorders, or associated symptoms that span diagnostic categories.

An individual child's longitudinal history may reveal this increasing complexity of symptoms. Rarely, however, does one have the opportunity in clinical practice to observe a child's development from the onset of the behavioral problem. Instead, the psychiatrist sees children at a point in time when their problems have already become sufficiently troublesome to be brought to professional attention. The psychiatrist must then use whatever evidence is available to assess the origin and course of the specific disorder.

The behavioral history reflects the interaction between a child's personality attributes and the significant features of his intrafamilial and extrafamilial environment. This interaction gives rise to stresses and strains. How the child deals with them depends upon his temperamental reactive pattern and the attitude of the persons who have meaningful relations with him. Stress in itself is not an inevitable cause of disturbed behavior. Sometimes, even a difficult demand, such as toilet training in some children, will be a healthy stimulus insofar as it leads the child to increased control over his environment. The crucial factor is the consonance of the demand with the child's behavioral style and abilities. When a child is confronted with excessive stress or demands that he cannot master in terms of either his temperamental reactions or his cognitive or physical abilities, maladaptive functioning may result. Obviously, what is stressful or dissonant for one child may not be so for another with different characteristics and abilities. It thus becomes necessary, when considering the various behavior difficulties of children, to relate them to specific interactive processes.

Some behavior reactions, although they create problems, are so transitory or slight that they may be considered a part of normal maturation. For example, sleep disturbances during an illness and for a brief period afterward are not unusual, nor is fear of dogs for weeks after a frightening experience with an animal. In the same category of normal behavior are minor annoying traits which children develop as appropriate reactions to a particular individual. A youngster may have a moderate tantrum whenever his grandmother refuses to grant his wishes because he knows from experience that she cannot bear to see him cry and will alter her decision. But the same youngster may behave reasonably with other persons who are not so easily swayed.

Other behaviors which appear abnormal may represent the temperamental attributes of a child. Some children who seem to display fears and anxiety when confronted with new situations may, in reality, be evidencing one aspect of their characteristic slowness to warm up. Similarly, a very persistent or a very distractible child may present various management problems in the face of learning demands. The behavior must be analyzed in terms of the child's history. One must be careful not to confuse what is normal and characteristic for one child with what may be a pathologic state in another of different reactivity.

Normal behavior reactions, when perpetuated, may become behavior disorders. For example, a child who has had a series of frightening experiences may become fearful of *any* new situation or change of plans, or he may develop phobic reactions.

Reactive Behavior Disorders

When reactions to environmental events, though maladaptive, are still flexible enough so that a change in the environment will suffice to alter the behavior, the disorder may be considered reactive.

In most cases, the disorder is limited to one or more specific areas of life but does not pervade other aspects of the child's functioning. Thus, a youngster who has a sleep problem may be learning to capacity in school and enjoying normal peer relationships. The particular symptoms are often determined by environmental influences. Parents and teachers make demands that reflect their own standards and values. If these demands are inappropriate to a child's capacities or previously developed behavior patterns, excessive stress may result. The child may begin to show maladaptive reactions in the specific functional areas where the demands are most persistent.

The behavioral response to an excessive or dissonant demand will depend upon the child's specific pattern of temperamental traits. For example, if a child who is slow to warm up is pressured by his parents to become immediately involved in new situations, he will often show withdrawal reactions of mild intensity. He may hide behind his mother when taken into a friend's home or may quietly and quickly retreat to the sidelines when taken to a new playground. On the other hand, if a difficult child of high intensity is confronted with the same demands in similar situations, he will often protest loudly and vigorously, and may even have a tantrum. One slow-to-warm up child who once got lost in a large department store when shopping with her mother developed a reactive separation anxiety and became quite clinging in new environments. But another child who tended to approach rather than withdraw from new experiences and warmed-up quickly had such a good time when she couldn't find her mother in the store that she has tried to get herself lost on every subsequent shopping expedition.

Treatment efforts in reactive behavior disorders are directed toward modification of the environment, with full awareness that in each case the child's reaction pattern is an important determinant of the most constructive approach to handling. Parent guidance is a useful therapeutic approach in these instances.

By making the parents his allies and showing them that they have not been "bad" parents, but that their methods have not been optimal for this particular child, the psychiatrist can often win their support in carrying out a corrective program of changed handling. Once they have been shown concretely how their methods of management have contributed to excessive stress and symptom formation, many parents can institute changes in their behavior which lead to amelioration of the child's symptoms and marked improvement in his overall functioning.

Neurotic Behavior Disorders

A child's defensive reactions may become so fixed and rigid that they cannot be altered simply by modification of the environment. In some cases, the initial appearance of a symptom causes a worsening of the child-environment interaction from which it has derived. A child's reactive behavior disorder may be so poorly handled, or he may be subjected to such a rapid succession of traumatic situations, that he begins to perceive events in terms of his distorted picture of the world around him. For example, one youngster became terrified of the street-corner Santa Clauses who appeared at Christmas time. It was impossible to explain this phobic reaction until an inadvertent remark showed the connection between his fears of Santa Claus and his fears of dying. During the previous Christmas season, the boy's grandfather and another important male figure had died. The traumas, one on top of the other, were too much for the child and led him to associate dying with Santa Claus.

Such a child may become incapable of reacting appropriately to a different environmental situation. Moreover, in his interactions with the environment, his defensive behavior may impinge on others and, in turn, create reactions which are in keeping with his distorted concept of people, thus reinforcing this concept. A youngster who is convinced that the world is a hostile place in which he must always defend himself is likely to have a chip on his shoulder in any peer relationships. A close decision in a baseball game, a playmate's accidental brushing against him, or playful name-calling may make him respond with a burst of fury. This reaction naturally mobilizes the hostility of the other children, who then proceed to treat him in the way he feared and indeed expected to be treated. Confirmation of this notion that everyone is out to "get" him reinforces his behavior, which is initially based on the idea that the best defense is attack. The same thing may be true of the timid child who makes no overtures and is therefore left out of group activities, or the little conniver who oversteps the boundary of what is acceptable among his peers and is rejected by them. In such situations, behavioral traits may become fixed and self-perpetuating.

Behavior disorders which are so rigid and severe that they are not modifiable within the ordinary exigencies of daily life may be considered neurotic. Treatment of neurotic behavior disorders requires a combined attack on the environment and the behavioral pattern. Because of the neurotic attitudes underlying the repetitive behavior pattern, direct treatment of the child is usually indicated. In some cases, however, if the parents can be truly objective and conscientious in maintaining remedial measures over an extended period of time, it is possible to modify the neurotic behavior pattern and the neurotic attitudes underlying it without direct treatment of the child.

Obviously, the best way to treat neurotic behavior disorders is by prevention. This calls for the appropriate handling of reactive disorders at their inception, while they can still be reversed, and before the fixed behavioral pattern characteristic of neurotic behavior disorders has been established.

The symptoms of a neurotic behavior disorder, like those of a reactive behavior disorder, reflect the specific child-environment interaction. Another important determinant of symptom formation is the developmental level of the child. Clinical observations indicate that in preschool children symptoms are expressed predominantly in overt behavior and action, whereas in older children they reflect complex subjective states, attitudes, distorted self images, and psychodynamic patterns of defense. This shift from action to ideation in symptoms parallels the change that occurs with normal maturation. These findings suggest that one should examine the dynamics of symptom formation and elaboration without invoking hypotheses about complex underlying motivational states in every case of disordered behavior in young children. At the same time, however, one must be wary of adopting a simple conditioned reflex model to explain all symptom evolution in older children in whom ideation, symbolic representation and abstraction play increasingly important roles.

One possible symptom of neurotic behavior disorders, sexual activity, merits special consideration. Parental concern about the sexual activity of children of all ages is common, but in some instances it is ill-founded and based on misinterpretation. Despite extensive writing on the normality of childhood expressions of sexuality, myths and folklore about the harmful consequences of sex play still persist. They account for children's guilt feelings about masturbation and sex play, and for a wide variety of misapprehensions among young and old about resultant castration, brain rot, "going crazy" and general "badness."

Moreover, exploration which is only accidentally or incidentally focused on the genital area is sometimes misconstrued as sexual. There is no cause to worry about the nine month old boy who grabs his penis if he is not given the powder box or a toy to play with when he is being diapered; he merely wants to hold something in his hands. Five year olds who undress to "play doctor" and take temperature with a "pretend thermometer" are usually not focusing on the genitals as a specific pleasure organ. The youngsters who on a few occasions indulge in sex play as a group may be exploring this area in the same healthy way that they explore other parts of their bodies.

Some children, however, manifest compulsive sexual activity, most commonly compulsive masturbation, as a symptom of a neurotic behavior disorder. The extent to which masturbation is hidden or disguised is directly related to the overt disapproval of masturbation shown by adults and the child's own level of social awareness. A very young child may be unaware of the element of strong social disapproval, but one who is masturbating openly after the age of five or six should ordinarily be aware of the pronounced social attitude toward this behavior. If he is not, such grave detachment from reality suggests serious pathology.

Compulsive masturbation is an expression of anxiety and poor interpersonal relationships. Some children can relax and fall asleep at night only after they have masturbated to a climax of sorts. Their difficulty lies in the tension produced by daytime events and relationships, and this tension must be reduced if their compulsive behavior is to be ameliorated. Other children masturbate at intervals during the day in various ways, by manipulation with their hands or objects, by rocking back and forth while seated with their feet tucked under their genitals, or by rubbing against chair arms or table corners.

To assess the severity and meaning of the symptom, it is necessary to examine the timing and duration of the compulsive activity, to discover whether it is preferred to social activity and what the degree of compulsion is, and to undertake a total review of the child's activities and personality.

Many parents find it difficult to spell out social expectations in the sexual area without, on the one hand, being so permissive that the child is ill-prepared for social taboos or, on the other, so punitive that anxiety is fostered. If parents are unable to convey the idea that the desire for privacy in the sexual area is not identical with the feeling of shame, it is no wonder that their children cannot make this distinction. The parent who can make clear to the six year old that nose-picking is not intrinsically bad but is nevertheless not an approved public act is often unable to get the same idea across in regard to masturbation or public exposure of the genital area.

Children who have witnessed adult sexual intercourse often become confused or sexually aroused, or they entirely misinterpret what they have seen. The child who has been subjected to direct sexual stimulation by an adult will have reactions of fear, sexual arousal or confusion about the sexual role of adults. The impact of such situations depends on the child's total adjustment to the event. At times, the commotion of the subsequent inquiry, if the event is discovered and the child is repeatedly questioned, may be even more traumatic than what actually happened. Chronic sexual exploitation of a child by an adult may be the basis for pronounced and stubborn maladjustment of the victim in adulthood.

Neurosis

Adult neurosis has its roots in the neurotic reactions of childhood and represents organized reactions of anxiety or of defense against anxiety. Childhood neurosis is relatively rare, perhaps because of the immaturity of the child's personality, or, to put it another way, because the child is still in the process of maturation and his neurotic reactions have not yet had time to become organized. On the basis of this time-element concept, it is easy to see why the incidence of neurosis is greater in adolescence than in childhood.

Although some attention has specifically been paid to childhood neuroses, most authors have applied the theoretic concepts worked out for adults directly to children, with little or no fundamental changes. In general, too, the approach of each psychiatrist has been a direct reflection of his theoretic orientation. These predispositions have been polarized in the positions taken by classical psychoanalysis and certain forms of learning theory with regard to the etiology of neurotic behavior. Contemporary psychoanalytic theory continues to be preoccupied with motives, as is shown by its search for the sources of psychopathologic phenomena in underlying purposes and conceptualized goals and aims. In contrast, Eysenck (1965) and other learning therapists deny the existence of underlying motivational states and declare that neurosis is, pure and simple, a conditioned maladaptive behavior.

To attribute elaborate motivational mechanisms to a young child is merely confusing if a simpler explanation in terms of a dissonant child-environment interaction can account for all the facts. In the older child, however, it may be necessary to invoke such motivational states when efforts to explain the behaviors in terms of simple mechanisms are inadequate.

While the question of motives has aroused much heated discussion, the role of anxiety in the origin and development of neuroses has been less controversial. No matter whether anxiety is defined as subjective distress or as autonomic reactions to painful stimuli, many theorists view neurotic symptoms as a technique for reducing anxiety and insulating an individual from it. And, in the connection that is usually made between anxiety and symptom, it is generally assumed that if there were no antecedent anxiety there would be no symptoms.

Contrary to these formulations, however, have been the findings of the New York Longitudinal Study (Thomas, 1968). In the children studied, anxiety was not evident prior to symptom development. Rather, it developed during the evolution of the child's behavior disorder as a secondary phenomenon, a consequence rather than a cause of symptom development and expression. Once the anxiety did appear, of course, it substantially influenced the dynamics of the child's functioning and the subsequent course of his behavior.

Our clinical and research data contradict another common assumption of those who view symptoms as purposively developed to reduce anxiety and conflict: the theory that symptom removal will result either in a rise in anxiety, in increased disorganization of functioning, or in the substitution of new symptoms for old. We have frequently used parent guidance as a therapeutic approach, with the aim of eliminating a child's symptoms. When this treatment method has been successful, we have found that there were concurrent and continuing positive effects on functioning and that no overt anxiety or substitutive symptoms developed.

Some of the neurotic reaction patterns of childhood represent, on an immature level, the neuroses of adulthood. Specific symptoms of adult neuroses—phobias, anxiety reactions, compulsions and fears—occur as specific neurotic traits in childhood. Youngsters may have phobias about animals, heights, open or closed spaces, people of a given appearance, certain kinds of clothing. They may experience anxiety reactions when riding in cars and trains, when separated from the mother or another member of the family, or in a host of other situations. They may develop compulsions to write or touch things a certain number of times, step on or avoid sidewalk cracks, arrange their clothing in an exact pattern at bed time, wash their hands continually, ask repetitious questions; and they often have fears about dying, growing up or being kidnaped. These anxiety and obsessive-compulsive neuroses permit the child to have a certain degree of freedom: so long as he can maintain his symbolic acts and avoid those things to which he has a phobic response, he is comfortable and feels fine. And, insofar as others cooperate with him, he may stay symptom-free. In such cases, the personality organization of the child has arrived at the point where he can respond as an adult does.

The child's age should be kept in mind, however, before concluding that a particular symptom is pathologic. The specific behavior may represent realization of dependency, exploration of the incompletely comprehended laws governing the environment, or misapprehension about cause and effect relationships based on the accidental and temporary juxtaposition of two events. The symptom should be designated as a neurotic trait only if it is clearly inappropriate for the child's age or if its expression usurps the place of normal relationships in the child's life.

The neurosis of conversion hysteria is found in prepuberty and adolescence. Almost any organ may be involved. It may take the form of paralysis or loss of sensation in one of the extremities, or it may appear as abdominal complaints. Sometimes the abdominal symptoms are severe enough to require hospitalization for a complete diagnostic work-up, and often the only indication that a laparotomy should not be performed is the absence of a high white blood cell count. Psychologic investigation may then reveal intense conflict in which ambivalent strivings and fears are evenly balanced. The somatic symptoms frequently provide a respite from the intolerable battle of such contending forces.

Psychosomatic symptoms also occur in children. Examples are the morning nausea or diarrhea of a child who is distressed or in conflict about his school situation, or the onset of an attack of asthma or neurodermatitis after an intense episode of sibling rivalry.

The diagnosis of conversion hysteria or of psychosomatic disturbance should not be made by a process of elimination. The absence of clear organic findings is not by itself sufficient evidence of conversion hysteria, although it should be a signal for investigating this possibility. Similarly, the absence of a clear-cut organic etiology does not automatically identify psychosomatic disease. The diagnosis must be based on a clear psychodynamic formulation which explains the symptoms in terms of underlying conflicts.

Occasionally, an apparent adolescent neurosis is the precursor of a schizophrenic process. Somatic complaints that appear to indicate conversion hysteria may be superseded by ideas of reference, clear delusions, pervasive anxiety, paranoid ideation or other symptoms pointing inexorably to a picture of adolescent schizophrenia. In a compulsion neurosis, obsessive thoughts may at first seem to respond to psychotherapy, only to reappear later with other symptoms of schizophrenia.

In such cases we do not know whether a neurosis has become transformed into schizophrenia or whether the disorder was undiagnosed schizophrenia in the first place. Findings have been cited in support of each view, but we do not as yet have sufficient knowledge to settle the argument. We can only say with certainty that when a well-defined neurosis is present before puberty or in early adolescence, the psychiatrist should be alert to the possibility of more serious morbidity later on.

Neurotic Character Disorders

The defensive patterns of neurotic behavior disorders may become so thoroughly integrated into the personality structure that they have to be regarded as characterologic. The child with a neurotic character disorder has more generalized anxiety and/or more distortion of interpersonal relationships than a child with a neurosis. His neurotic functioning is rigidified, and he no longer is really troubled by it. The youngster's distorted impressions of other people's motives, attitudes and conduct cause him to behave in such a way as to engender unfavorable responses from those around him. In turn, these responses generate further neurotically defensive behavior in a vicious cycle.

The distinction between neurotic character disorder and neurotic behavior disorder is based primarily on a judgment of the degree of severity. The greater consistency and intensity of the distorted perception in a neurotic character disorder results in a poorer prognosis, even if an intensive attack is made on both the underlying neurotic attitudes and the environment, because the child generally has little or no motivation for change. Although unhappy about his situation, he does not see his own behavior as contributing to it. Some event or some constructive relationship, however, may illuminate for the child the self-destructiveness of his ways of relating to his environment and this may provide motivation for change. A psychotherapeutic attempt will then have a better chance of success.

Sociopathic Character Disorder

The character disturbance known as sociopathic personality was long regarded as constitutional, and the diagnosis "constitutional psychopath" was used so frequently that it became a psychiatric grab bag. Psychiatrists today are more aware of the effects of environmental forces in shaping the sociopathic personality, and they are more careful to distinguish between this disturbance and other diagnostic categories.

The individual with a sociopathic personality is characterized by impulsive behavior, inability to plan ahead and absence of empathy with the feelings and needs of others. He commits destructive acts without any sense of guilt or pang of conscience.

A number of studies have suggested that there may be a relationship between inconsistent and unstable care in the first two years of life and the character structure of the sociopathic personality, particularly in regard to the lack of development of object relationships. Foundlings brought up in institutions and cared for by frequently changing personnel, infants moved from one foster home to another, children in their own homes cared for by a succession of mother substitutes seemed with impressive regularity to develop into sociopathic personalities. On the basis of these studies, it has been suggested that this disturbance is not constitutional but is acquired as a result of a particular combination of life experiences. On the other hand, as noted earlier, some children with unstable earlier environments do not develop this type of personality, whereas one also finds sociopaths who come from stable living circumstances.

The differential diagnosis of a child with a sociopathic personality may cover a wide range of possibilities. For example, a child growing up in an area where delinquency is prevalent may indulge in antisocial acts with no apparent anxiety as a way of adjusting to the dog-eat-dog mores of his environment and of meeting his social needs for companionship. An examination of his relationships with members of his family may reveal a normal ability to form object relationships and an adequate sense of social responsibility. With this history, the child cannot be diagnosed as a sociopath. A youngster whose behavior resembles that of a sociopathic personality may present evidence of anxiety, fears or phobias of various kinds; these are indications of a psychodynamic process other than sociopathic personality.

In adolescence, there may be a picture of a sociopathic personality with no suggestion that this disorder was present in the pre-adolescent history. The change may be due to the strong influence of peer groups in this age period. This may be considered an adjustment reaction of adolescence. On the other hand, the appearance of sociopathic behavior in adolescence may be the first symptom of schizophrenia. It is often difficult to differentiate between adolescent schizophrenia and sociopathic personality because in both disorders there may be failure of adequate reality testing, impulsive behavior without guilt feelings, inability to learn from disaster and absence of concern about the effects of behavior on others. In both conditions the prognosis is poor, whether or not treatment is attempted. To make the diagnosis, further longitudinal study of the adolescent's behavior over a period of time may be necessary. Formal psychologic testing may clarify the nature of the thought disorder.

Associated Symptoms

In addition to the specific categories discussed above, there is a group of symptoms that may occur in a variety of psychiatric disorders.

Enuresis

Diurnal enuresis is comparatively rare, but nocturnal enuresis occurs so frequently that provisions for handling it are made as a matter of course in summer camps.

It is usually assumed that the child who wets his bed often after he is three years old is suffering from anxiety or tension of an unhealthy psychologic nature. However, before initiating treatment on the basis of this assumption, one must clearly determine that the symptom is caused by psychodynamic stress.

Obviously, one first checks on the possibility of an organic cause, particularly disease of the urinary tract or a systemic illness which may account for the poor bladder control. With these causes ruled out, it is necessary to investigate the possibility of an "irritable bladder." In this condition, imbalance of sympathetic-parasympathetic functioning decreases conscious control of the sphincter, especially in deep sleep. When this cause is identified, there is often a familial history of enuresis.

One must also assess the physical set-up in which the child lives as well as the attitudes of his social group toward bedwetting. In a "cold water" flat where the toilet is in an outside, dimly lit, unheated hall, going to the toilet is an uncomfortable and frightening journey for the child. Under such conditions enuresis may be a natural adjustment to the physical environment rather than a psychologic reaction, such as an expression of hostility toward the mother. Moreover, in the social group to which the child belongs, bedwetting may not be considered a problem but merely what is expected at his age.

If enuresis is the only symptom in an otherwise reasonably well-adjusted child, it probably does not represent conflict or other psychologic difficulty. Conditioning, either by toileting the child at regular times or by some mechanical device, may suffice to clear up the problem. On the other hand, enuresis that is one of a number of behavioral symptoms is quite likely to be psychogenic.

It may be an expression of fear and fright. It may be an indication of deep hostility toward the parents which cannot be openly expressed. There may be the added element of pleasure from the stream of warm water on the inner surface of the thighs. Unconcern over bedwetting may be but one element in the general picture of the sociopathic child who is without any idea of impulse control. Finally, enuresis may be directly related to a situation of specific stress. For example, the child who wets on Sunday through Thursday nights—the nights preceding school days—and never on the nights preceding weekends and other school holidays may be reacting to extreme stress in his school life.

Enuresis of psychologic origin will respond to treatment insofar as the underlying psychologic problem responds to treatment. Before and during treatment, attempts to control enuresis by punishment or humiliation should be avoided, since such measures will only intensify the underlying psychologic difficulty.

Whatever its cause, enuresis is generally the source of further disturbances. The child who wets is ashamed to let his friends know about his weakness. He therefore hesitates to spend the night at their homes or have them in his home overnight, and he refuses to go to camp or on overnight hikes. He may have been subjected to shaming and punishment in an effort to train him, and this may have created further difficulties. Sometimes the youngster covers up his feelings of helplessness by bravado, saying, "I do it on purpose. I can stop if I want to, but I don't want to." His bravado in this situation may well carry over into other areas.

Stuttering

It is frequently assumed that stuttering is entirely psychogenic. In some cases, however, stuttering has a physiologic base, and in others the cause cannot be identified.

As S. T. Orton (1937) observed, a child who is trained to a handedness opposite to his spontaneous development may respond with stuttering. When such a child is changed back to the naturally dominant hand for writing and eating, stuttering often disappears. In some instances, stuttering appears to be present when there is a confusion of a developmental nature in cerebral dominance. The speech difficulty may also occur as a result of organic brain pathology.

In stuttering of psychologic origin, the dynamics of the causation may be in any diagnostic category. The stuttering child may be afraid to be assertive, particularly in verbal expression. He may have this fear because his thoughts are so violent that he anticipates retaliation, or he may picture himself as small and helpless in a hostile and dangerous world. He may have obsessive thoughts which he seeks to keep from voicing through stuttering. Some children who stutter do not have behavioral or adjustment difficulties; their behavior in all other respects may be normal. Thus it appears that there is a classification of stuttering which we do not understand. For stutterers in this group, psychotherapy has not offered direct relief. Speech therapy may be helpful. In many cases, the stuttering becomes less prominent or even disappears when it is treated as a speech handicap. During treatment an attempt should be made to limit the effects of the handicap in its interference with the youngster's functioning, and to keep it from becoming the nucleus of reactions of shame, lack of confidence, feelings of worthlessness and defensiveness.

School Phobia

Certain abnormal reactions to school may be of such a disruptive nature that they are now commonly termed *school phobia*. This phenomenon may occur either during a child's initial school experience or after several years of apparently good adjustment at school. In the latter case, a detailed scrutiny of the initial school adjustment may reveal evidences of earlier anxieties which the child appeared to have overcome.

School phobia must be differentiated from nonattendance at school because of lack of interest, shame at poor academic performance or involvement in delinquent activities. It also must be distinguished from the withdrawal reactions of a child who is temperamentally slow to warm up when he first begins school. A true phobic reaction is an expression of intense anxiety in the school situation from which the child protects himself by withdrawing from the school. School phobia is not a diagnosis in itself; it is a symptom that may be found in almost any diagnostic category.

The normal child who is frightened by some event in the school building or whose initial school experience is with a shouting, punitive teacher may have a short-lived phobic reaction to school. If this reaction persists but can be eliminated by a change in the environment—another teacher, another school or some other appropriate change—the difficulty is in the category of reactive behavior disorders. In such cases, school phobia may be the solitary symptom.

If the school difficulty is one among many symptoms, the total evaluation may lead to a diagnosis of neurotic behavior or neurotic character disorder. Or, the fundamental disturbance may be an anxiety neurosis, an obsessive-compulsive neurosis, or conversion hysteria. The hypermotility and short attention span of the child with cerebral dysfunction or the sensitivity of the physically handicapped child may result in phobic reactions to a teacher's reprimands. Anxiety in the schoolroom may be the first presenting symptom of a disorder that is severe enough to direct attention to a diagnosis of schizophrenia.

Usually, school phobia is one among a group of difficulties that form a pattern pointing toward some basic dysfunction. The child and his family may not even recognize that school is the locus of anxiety. They may be concerned about nausea or abdominal aches and cramps. The child may have dizzy spells, vague dreads, worry about the mother's safety and other complaints. After careful questioning, it generally becomes clear that he is free from these symptoms on weekends and school holidays and that the difficulties always occur in school and make school attendance agony for him. The youngster may also worry that the teacher will not allow him to leave the classroom in time if he says that he is going to vomit, or will not permit him to go home if he says he feels ill.

Whatever the nature of the organ representation of anxiety, clues must be sought in the child's general behavior under stress. Is the stress fear of separation from the mother? If so, one will find other indications of separation anxiety: reluctance to go to other children's homes to play, scenes at night when the parents go out and inability to fall asleep until the mother returns, insistence that she remain with him while he plays outdoors. Is the stress fear of failure? If so, the child will not only show panic about school assignments; he will also have low frustration-tolerance, be a poor loser and be unable to take criticism gracefully. If the teacher is a symbol of dreaded authority figures, this reaction shows up in other phases of the child's life. If other children are symbols of hostility, he avoids playing with groups, and he makes comments expressing derogation or fear of his peers. Is the school phobia caused by the child's inability to function in a situation which he cannot dominate and control? If so, we will find that he rules the roost at home and that away from home he tries to boss his playmates or has tantrums.

In sum, school phobia must be assessed in terms of the child's out-of-school behavior and treated on the basis of whatever findings are disclosed by careful examination.

Homosexuality

It is difficult to classify the homosexual child in terms of one of the diagnostic categories discussed above. There may or may not be a clear underlying neurotic basis for the child's tendency to identify with the opposite sex; if there is, homosexuality may be a secondary issue that is likely to disappear if the neurotic difficulty is cleared up.

A little boy who has observed that in his family his sister is accepted and he is rejected may attempt to find a place for himself by identifying with his more favorably treated sibling. Similarly, the little girl who finds that her world gives no prestige to females may seek a place in the sun by identifying with the males in her environment. The child of either sex with a strong attachment to the parent of the opposite sex and a destructive relationship with the parent of the same sex may respond with mixed sexual identification. Confusion in sexual identification arising from these and many other neurotic patterns is modifiable to the extent that the underlying neurotic problem is modifiable.

A child whose behavior runs counter to the social clichés for his or her sex is sometimes incorrectly considered to be homosexual. A little boy may be gentle or passive, and a little girl may be aggressive. In neither case should the child be described as homosexual merely on the basis of personality traits.

A reciprocal relationship between homosexuality and schizophrenia has been reported in which a successful "cure" of homosexuality has been followed by a psychotic breakdown or a psychotic episode has gone into remission following a homosexual adjust-

ment. Both homosexuality and schizophrenia have been ascribed
to the parental constellation of a passive father and an aggressive
mother. This particular combination, however, has been accused
of nurturing many other kinds of psychiatric disorders, and it is
questionable whether it can be considered specific for any of them.

Above and beyond these types of cases, however, there remains
a very large group of homosexuals whose disturbed sexual development is due to obscure reasons.

Suicide

Threats of suicide are made by children of all ages. Although
they are usually hostile gestures designed to hurt someone in the
environment, they should always be taken seriously and evaluated
carefully. The child who swallows the full contents of a bottle of
aspirin with few ill effects may on another occasion take something
that has more tragic results.

The young child does not have a clear idea of the finality of
death. Like Tom Sawyer, he pictures himself watching adults'
reactions as they view his lifeless body, and at the same time he
makes plans for what he is going to do in life. When a child says,
"I'm going to kill myself," or, "I wish I wasn't born," his statements should be assessed in the light of his general adjustment and
how the parents reacted overtly the first time he made such a
statement. Careful consideration must be given to the secondary
gains and elements of "blackmail" in such threats.

Children who find that suicide threats evoke great parental
solicitation make constant use of this device. In attempting to
avoid this outcome, parents should be helped to make a distinction
between changes in handling an unhappy child to give him greater
security and letting themselves be ruled by the child's suicide
threats. If a child uses such threats successfully in his early years,
he may later on have so great a need to tyrannize and dominate
that it may be dangerous to call his bluff when he threatens suicide.
In his intense drive to maintain the power he has exercised successfully as a younger child, he may do something that results in
personal injury or death.

Suicide threats made by preadolescents and adolescents when they
are in a depressed state may indicate serious pathology. As with

adults, the difficult problem is to assess the probability of acting out. It is generally preferable to resolve the issue without hospitalization, but this is not always possible, and residential treatment may be required. The therapist's primary initial responsibility is to make certain that the suicide threats are not carried out and to preserve the patient's life.

Compulsive Eating and Anorexia Nervosa

The symptoms of compulsive eating with resultant obesity and compulsive refusal to take adequate nourishment, or anorexia nervosa, are seen in the practice of child psychiatry. Of the two, compulsive eating is far more common.

The roles of mother and giver of food are interwoven in the child's first year of life when feeding means warmth, being held, and a general feeling of pleasure. As the child grows older he responds to the mother's expressed concern, or lack of concern, about his eating and her general attitude toward him. For example, children of neglectful mothers are usually not "picky" eaters, and they may take food from the refrigerator in excess of their food intake needs. On the other hand, the child whose mother focuses on his eating habits and expresses constant concern about them learns that refusal to eat is a potent weapon against his mother and that eating is a gift he makes to her. A hostility-dependency relationship develops, with a battle of wills between mother and child. The intensity of this conflict is reflected in the battle of the breakfast, lunch and dinner table.

When food becomes for the child a symbol of love and affection, he turns to compulsive eating if he feels bereft of love. He may actually be deprived of love; or he may be insatiable in his demands for attention and feel deprived because of sibling rivalry or other psychologic problems of relationship. If the youngster eats excessively and becomes obese, the mother may try to limit his food intake; the child may then submit with concealed or overt rage, he may eat more food on the sly, or he may steal money to buy candy.

Although hostility is often the dominant hidden motivation in compulsive eating, less severe forms of this symptom may also be expressions of anxiety attacks of varying duration—a day, several days, or even weeks. The secondary gains need to be considered.

One is the easily obtained gain of controlling the actions of significant persons who give in to the child through fear of precipitating
another attack. Another is escape from situations that produce
anxiety. For example, if the child's unattractively obese appearance
is a good "alibi" for nonparticipation in some anxiety-provoking
activity, the motivation for retaining the symptom may become even
more powerful than the drive to obtain release from it.

Anorexia nervosa is a descriptively clear syndrome which appears
in girls, usually during their early adolescence. Typically, a physically healthy but overweight individual voluntarily goes on a reducing diet and then continues to limit her food intake far beyond
the original intention. Progressive weight loss may reach the point
of emaciation and even death. In many cases, the patient is a girl
whose mother had made a big issue of eating habits. During the
child's infancy, the mother may have pressed her to eat, and then,
during preadolescence, exhorted her to cut down her intake so she
would lose weight. A hostile, dependent relationship develops between mother and child. The problems that had entered into the
excessive eating are transferred to the dieting. With the successful
attainment of slimness, the diet becomes a compulsive expression of
hostility. The mother wins a Pyrrhic victory—a skeleton-like child.
The youngster is caught in a self-destructive situation in which she
is unable to abandon a potent weapon against the mother, even if
she destroys herself by using it.

The mother-child hostility is almost never the sole psychiatric
factor operating in cases of anorexia nervosa. The reducing diet is
usually begun by the girl on her own volition as she becomes aware
that her figure is distasteful both to herself and to other persons.
This awareness typically occurs at puberty and coincides with a
general change from a childish to a womanly figure. While menstruation itself is not usually a precipitating traumatic event, the
history almost always reveals some definable situation in which female
maturity was equated with danger. The child may have had a close
relative who died during pregnancy or delivery, or she may have
some other painful association with marriage. The severe diet may
then give the youngster not merely the socially acceptable aim of
acquiring the type of feminine figure that is more favored in our
culture, but also the unconscious aim of halting adult growth and
retaining her prepubertal safety.

Anorexia nervosa may occur in almost all the psychiatric categories described earlier in this chapter. Some youngsters, apart from the specific syndrome, seem to be quite normal in their previous history and current functioning, with adequate peer and family relationships, successful academic careers and normal affective capacities. In others, the syndrome accompanies a reactive problem in which other symptoms may also appear; in still others, a neurotic pattern exists or the girl may be psychotic, mentally retarded or have cerebral dysfunction.

SELECTED REFERENCES

Eysenck, H. J., and Rachman, S.: *The Causes and Cures of Neurosis: An Introduction to Modern Behavior Therapy Based on Learning Theory and the Principles of Conditioning.* San Diego, Knapp, 1965.

Finch, S. M.: *Fundamentals of Child Psychiatry.* New York, W. W. Norton, 1960.

Glaser, K.: Masked depression in children and adolescents. *Amer. J. Psychother.* 21:565-574, 1967.

Kahn, J. H., and Nursten, J. P.: School refusal: a comprehensive view of school phobia and other failures of school attendance. *Amer. J. Orthpsychiat.* 32:707, 1962.

Kanner, L.: *Child Psychiatry.* Springfield, Ill., Charles C Thomas, 1957.

Lesser, L. I., Ashenden, B. J., Debuskey, M., and Eisenberg, L.: Anorexia nervosa in children. *Amer. J. Orthopsychiat.* 30:572-580, 1960.

Orton, S.: *Reading, Writing and Speech Problems in Children.* New York, W. W. Norton, 1937.

Shaw, C. R.: *The Pychiatric Disorders of Childhood.* New York, Appleton-Century-Crofts, 1966.

_____, and Schelkun, R.: Suicidal behavior in children. *Psychiatry,* 28:157, 1965.

Thomas, A., Chess, S., and Birch, H. G.: *Temperament and Behavior Disorders in Children.* New York, New York University Press, 1968.

12. Childhood Schizophrenia and Psychosis

CHILDHOOD SCHIZOPHRENIA is a frequently diagnosed but inadequately understood category of deviant behavior. Despite an abundance of theoretic views, its etiology remains obscure.

In the early days of psychiatry the condition was not identified, although 100 years ago Henry Maudsley (1867) devoted a chapter of his *Physiology and Pathology of the Mind* to insanity in child- • hood. Many children who would today be considered schizophrenic were once regarded as mental retardates or constitutional psychopaths. At the beginning of this century, Sante de Sanctis (1925) first described dementia praecox in adolescent children. In 1911, the term *schizophrenia* was introduced by Eugen Bleuler (1950), who observed that "With relatively accurate case histories, one can trace back the illness to childhood, or even to the first years of life, in at least five percent of the cases." American literature on this subject was launched by H. W. Potter (1933) with a report on an eleven year old boy who had begun to manifest symptoms of the disease at three and one-half years of age. Potter pointed out that schizophrenia before puberty was not so rare as was generally believed.

Theories of Childhood Schizophrenia

At first, the concept of schizophrenia was applied cautiously only to children whose behavior was extremely deviant. Thus Charles Bradley (1941), expressing the prevailing view in the early 1940's, maintained that for a positive diagnosis of schizophrenia to be made, the child had to be psychotic. Today, many psychiatrists reject the view that schizophrenic children invariably experience a psychotic break with reality.

Psychiatrists have also revised the formerly common opinion that a precondition for diagnosis is the prior existence of a period of normalcy. The earlier theory is reflected in Bradley's assertion that the child's disorder must have appeared "without known or obvious cause after a period in earlier life when he was *comparatively* free from mental disorder." This view was effectively challenged by Leo Kanner. In delineating the concept of early infantile autism, Kanner (1949) notes: "The great importance of the group which I have described as early infantile autism lies in the correction of the impression that a comparatively normal period of adjustment must precede the development of schizophrenia. Furthermore, this group shows that schizophrenic withdrawal can and does begin as early as in the diaper stage."

Many workers also agree with Kanner in rejecting the earlier theory that childhood schizophrenia represents a single entity. Kanner (1957) refers to "the schizophrenias of childhood" (it should be noted that Bleuler's classic work was titled *Dementia Praecox or the Group of Schizophrenias*). My own concept is that childhood schizophrenia is a behavioral syndrome that can derive from a number of etiologies which have not yet been completely identified. For such a concept the history of medicine offers impressive support. Time and again, syndromes that were once considered a single clinical disease have been subdivided into a number of entities with advances in knowledge of etiology.

Kanner's diagnostic designation of primary infantile autism has been widely accepted as a specific subgroup in the classification of childhood schizophrenia. The term is used to describe children who have a primary defect in their ability to respond affectively to their environment. Children with this disorder do not respond to the persons taking care of them. They do not cuddle, and they are more responsive to objects than to people. Along with this failure to react, they may not learn to talk and hence may resemble retarded or aphasic children.

As a result, one must be on guard against characterizing developmental aphasia or mental retardation as primary infantile autism. A diagnosis of autism cannot be based merely on deviation of affect. There must be some indication, no matter how sporadic or fleeting, that the child's capacity to form ideas is higher than that represented by his speech level. Autism cannot be conclusively postulated if the limitation of affect is consistent with the general picture of retarded ideation and speech level.

In addition to autism, the "symbiotic" type of childhood schizophrenia has been described by Margaret Mahler (1952). Some cases of schizophrenia, she believes, represent a symbiotic fusion of the egos of mother and child. The child is extremely clinging. He "melts into" the mother's body. Failing to make any differentiation between himself and the mother, he is unable to function as an independent entity. According to Mahler, both the symbiotic and autistic types are basically the result of pathologic mothering. While a constitutional predisposition is also postulated in this theory, the essential etiologic agent is the "schizophrenogenic" mother. Whether the child becomes autistic or symbiotic is determined by the stage of individuation (as described by psychoanalytic theory) at which the pathologic mothering occurs.

Other investigators, notably William Goldfarb (1961), have observed that many schizophrenic children have clearcut signs of neurologic pathology. With the development of more refined techniques of examination, neurologic damage is being identified in an increasing proportion of schizophrenic children. Follow-up studies have revealed the presence of convulsions and other neurologic disorders that were not originally present. The investigations of Mildred Creak (1963) have revealed neurologic lesions at autopsy.

There is growing evidence that children who are diagnosed as schizophrenic have some basic organic defect. Lauretta Bender was the first to emphasize the biologic nature of the disease. She regards the primary symptoms as being determined by biologic difficulty, with the secondary symptoms arising later as the child becomes aware of his basic difficulty and attempts to master it. Bender (1968) views childhood schizophrenia as a total organismic disorder characterized by a "lag in maturation" and the persistence of embryonic plasticity of the central nervous system: "The neurological hierarchy and control remain primitive, resembling in many aspects the organization of behavior found in the fetal stages of development." Among the secondary problems, Bender finds "disturbances in the body image, identity, and orientation to impersonal objects and forces from the outer world."

The genetic determination of both childhood and adult schizophrenia has been considered by various investigators, including Franz Kallman. Noting a high concordance rate in identical schizoid twins, Kallman (1956) suggests that "Children who display schizophrenic personality changes at an early age are distinguished not only by a specific vulnerability factor in the enzymatic range, but also by a general constitutional inability, or lowered ability, to control through compensatory activity this basic deficiency in the complex processes of growth and maturation."

Specific biochemical defects have been implicated by a number of investigators. Arnold Friedhoff (1967), for example, has identified an atypical amine in urine obtained from schizophrenic patients. Radioisotope studies indicate that "there may be a defect in biological transmethylation associated with schizophrenia." Further exploration and validation of such findings would obviously have important implications for the study of childhood schizophrenia.

Even if one cannot identify any specific organic damage, this may be because our present techniques for locating such defects are limited, not because the defects do not in fact exist. We are only at the beginning stage of biochemical and neurologic investigation of childhood schizophrenia.

But the organic aspect, in any event, cannot be considered in isolation. Its effect on the child's functioning is determined by interaction with the environment. To understand the specific features of pathologic behavior, one must examine in detail the simultaneous and interactive operation of organismic and environmental factors. Thus, if a child has a defective capacity to learn organized behavior patterns and social flexibility, he will become even more bewildered and show subsequent deviations in his behavior when faced with environmental demands that are not consonant with his needs and abilities.

An interactionist approach must take into full account all the influential factors in a situation. As an illustration, let us consider one of the basic findings in childhood schizophrenia, the inability of the child to make a meaningful interpersonal relationship. This phenomenon appears at a very early age and is one of the major diagnostic criteria. Those who take an organic approach would emphasize that the interpersonal defect is due to the child's maturational lag or, perhaps, his biochemical or neurologic defect. Variations in the intensity of the symptom would be related to variations in the degree of the lag or defect. On the other hand, environmentalists would attribute the interpersonal problem to some pathogenic influence of the parent, viewing the symptom as the direct result of this influence.

In contrast, the interactionist hypothesis is that the schizophrenic child's inability to establish a meaningful relationship with another human being reflects the interplay of two sets of factors. The first is the infant's fundamental difficulty in organizing and integrating incoming stimuli, whether the problem is due to a neurophysiologic or biochemical defect. But this difficulty is inseparable from a second, the fact that to an infant a human being represents a stimulus of enormous complexity and variability. When the child is confronted by another person, his basic difficulty is intensified by the heavy demands for processing novel stimuli. The infant's pathologic responses are not the direct result of either factor alone but of their interaction.

New kinds of behavioral symptoms appear as environmental demands become more complex. For instance, a four year old child who is given a toy truck to play with may limit his attention to the wheels, rolling them repetitiously with a finger. The limited nature of his play may be the sole symptom of abnormality so long as nobody tries to take the toy away, scolds him or attempts to interest him in another use of the toy. But by the time such a child is six years old, he may manifest behavior that is more obviously pathologic. In a classroom he may ask a set of repetitious questions, or he may scream if his accustomed seating arrangement is changed. At this later age, the child experiences numerous environmental demands that he use materials in ways that are beyond his competence. He is called upon to respond to individuals in a differentiated manner. He experiences a rapid building up of demands to which he cannot respond in an organized fashion. Moreover, since his attempts to meet these demands are likely to evoke scolding or teasing, anxiety may be added to the behavioral picture.

The behavioral characteristics of schizophrenic children have often been described in terms of disturbances in speech, motility, relationships with people and level of interest. Intensive anxiety reactions and great isolation may also be found, as well as evidence of early disturbance in eating and sleeping patterns and unusual receptor sensitivity.

In many cases it is extremely difficult to distinguish between mental deficiency and schizophrenia, as already noted in relation to autism. On the one hand, defective mental functioning may be one of the symptoms of schizophrenia; on the other hand, a behavior pattern that appears bizarre for the child's chronologic age—an indication of schizophrenia—is frequently found in the mentally defective child. In making the differential diagnosis, the child's behavior must be assessed in terms of his intellectual level. Intellectual functioning—as expressed in play, for example—that is uniformly below what may be expected at the child's chronologic age suggests retardation. But any indications of variability in intellectual functioning, any qualities that suggest a capacity to operate on a higher level, make the diagnosis of retardation less likely. The schizophrenic child shows some indications, whether fragmented or consistent, of intellectual functioning at or above the level expected for his age. Thus, a child's Goodenough drawing which indicates adequate comprehension of the human body would throw doubt on a diagnosis of retardation, even if the youngster's comprehension in other respects seems retarded. One should add, however, that retardation and schizophrenia may coexist as two separate entities in the same child.

Unfortunately, the history does not clear up these diagnostic issues: not all retarded children have a consistently slow development from birth, and not all schizophrenic children have a normal development up to the point at which symptoms of their illness appear. The histories of many retarded children report average ages, or even earlier than average ages, for sitting, standing, walking or the onset of speech. And the histories of schizophrenic children often reveal disturbances in speech, motility and sleep, and perhaps hyperirritability in early childhood and infancy. Furthermore, any of the behavior patterns and traits found in schizophrenic children may also be seen in children with organic disturbances or behavior disorders, and in normal children under certain circumstances. For example, a lack of interest in the environment may be caused by high fever or varying degrees of blindness or deafness. Similarly, intense pervasive interest in a single endeavor may indicate constructive preoccupation with a problem, or it may be a signal of organic brain disturbance, retardation or childhood schizophrenia. The diagnosis must therefore be based on an assessment of the essential characteristics of each disturbance, not on the superficial resemblances of the symptoms to those of one or another disease entity.

To determine the specific behavior characteristics of a group of fourteen schizophrenic children, Sulamith Wolff and I (1964) made an inductive analysis of detailed, systematically recorded information about the children's current behavior. We were interested in discovering aspects of behavior common to all the children as well as behavioral differences within the group.

The children were ranked according to a clinical impression of the severity of their illness. This impression was garnered through protocol interviews with the mothers, observations of the children, school records, and information about the family history, birth history, health and general development of each child. We also took into account the degree of emotional contact with others that the child could make and the amount of useful speech he had.

The distribution of abnormal behavior patterns indicated a continuum extending from the most severely affected children, who have no speech and only a small range of simple repetitive behavior, to the least severely affected who display useful (though abnormal) speech and a wider range of more complex behavior. Certain forms of abnormal behavior were common to all fourteen children, regardless of the severity of their illness. These included abnormalities of eye-to-eye contact, contributing to a clinical impression of emotional withdrawal; repetitive behavior, which appears to have no aim beyond the activity itself; abnormal communication of wishes; and failure to respond to clear-cut stimuli. Thirteen of the children showed unusual discriminative abilities in certain areas and obsessional patterns.

The similarity of symptoms does not imply that the etiology is the same in all cases or that there is necessarily a single disease process. One must attempt to be specific. It is not accurate to describe childhood schizophrenia in terms of a general affective withdrawal or a general failure to acquire the abstract attitude. Nor is it sufficient to characterize the disorder in terms of functioning at a generally lower level of development. Instead, the most characteristic quality of these children is their tendency to perform certain acts, appropriate for an earlier developmental stage or environmental context, in a repetitive and stereotyped manner long after the child's general development has reached a higher level of organization and the environmental situation has changed. It is as if patterns of behavior once evoked by specific stimuli continue to be elicited despite the profoundly altered context of the stimuli. While schizophrenic children resemble each other in the types of behavior affected by this distorting process (the way they look at other people, their motor behavior, their handling of objects), the behavioral acts themselves, particularly those acquired after infancy, bear the imprint of each child's individual life experiences.

Treatment

Concepts of etiology necessarily influence the approach to treatment. If the early parent-child relationship is viewed as primary, the therapy is directed toward correcting disturbance in this relationship. This approach emphasizes the development of a positive affective relationship with the therapist. Thus Mahler (1952) suggests that the autistic child be "lured out of his . . . shell with all kinds of devices such as music, rhythmic activities and pleasurable stimulation of his sense organs." In contrast, the symbiotic child must be left to test reality gradually at his own pace and, since he sees himself as fused with his mother, he must obtain a great deal of borrowed ego support from the therapist.

Adverse parental handling, however, does not in itself cause childhood schizophrenia. While rejected children have been found to have serious problems, schizophrenia is not statistically prominent among them. Beyond doubt, the schizophrenic child's relationship with his parents is difficult and frequently hostile. But careful perusal of the history often reveals that the beginning of aberrant behavior was noted as far back as the hospital newborn nursery. The seemingly adverse maternal handling may reflect the mother's despair at the unpredictability of the infant's reactions.

Bender (1968) has formulated general therapeutic principles in terms of her theory that the disturbance is essentially biologic and maturational. The child's lagging processes, she emphasizes, must be stimulated and his anxiety relieved. He must be helped to cope more successfully with internal and external tensions. Bender has advocated the use of electroshock or LSD in the treatment of schizophrenic children, but few workers would agree with this approach.

At the present level of our knowledge, we lack techniques for reversing whatever organic deviances may underlie schizophrenia. In the absence of such techniques, I believe that treatment depends upon an accurate assessment of the child-environment interaction. On the basis of such an assessment, the ,psychiatrist should define for the parents the optimum handling that might make it possible for their defective child to develop a repertoire of acceptable social responses, even if these are only mechanical. In order to minimize or reverse secondary behavior disturbances, the therapist should work out a plan for education that is realistically based on the child's ability to organize his behavior, as well as on his other capacities and qualities.

The fact that there may be a constitutional defect in childhood schizophrenia has sometimes been taken to mean that the child is born schizophrenic, with environmental influences providing only the milieu for the abnormal behavior. According to those who reason this way, treatment is useless since the constitutional factor is unmodifiable.

This attitude is not justified. The organic defect is not solely responsible. Careful study of the interaction between the biologically deviant infant and his environment may give clues to methods of preventing the development of the total schizophrenic picture.

It is productive to regard the schizophrenic child as a permanently handicapped youngster for whom psychotherapy is analogous to rehabilitation. Treatment should not be oriented to the same goal as that which would be set for handling a neurotic behavior disorder. Instead, as in the process of rehabilitating a physically handicapped individual, therapy requires a retraining in some functions, a training of other functions not previously involved to assume part of the burden, and a definition of situations in which outside help will be needed because they are clearly beyond the patient's capacity to handle by himself.

To achieve these goals, parent guidance is one procedure that may be effective. This approach aims to orient the parents to their child's abilities, disabilities and needs so that they can anticipate potential problem situations and deal with them in the best way possible. Let us assume that the schizophrenic child has incurred some damage, whether biochemical, neurologic, structural or perceptual, so that he is incapable of forming patterned responses in the normal way. The psychiatrist can help the parents understand what this means in terms of the child's present and future functioning. The parents need clear-cut advice about how to train the child to make full use of his abilities within the framework of his handicap.

Parents should be taught to present new learning demands deliberately and gradually, one small step at a time. They must be impressed with the importance of selecting carefully what should be taught, since a schizophrenic child will hold on tenaciously once he "gets" the pattern of behavior they are trying to teach him. A guidance approach that stresses the dangers of teaching too much at one time is helpful in building up parental awareness that the child's constitutional defect interferes with his ability to respond productively to the environment, to form patterns of behavior in response to environmental patterns, to learn in the usual manner. The youngster's handicap prevents him from giving full attention, in terms commensurate with his intellectual endowment, to the world around him.

In the attempt of schizophrenic children to master their environment we observe the intensification and prolongation of the usual modes of mastery—primary repetition, practice, and imitation. In their intensified forms, these modes appear as perseveration, compulsion, echolalia, echopraxia.

As many studies have indicated, the thoughts of schizophrenic children are not disconnected; rather, the unstated connections are dissimilar to those we expect and cannot be supplied by our empathetic completion of a stated word. For a normal child, we would complete the unstated connection and call the final product deep thinking, originality of ideas, unusual perspicacity. The schizophrenic child's deviation from the usual flow of ideas is usually described in such terms as autism, contamination, disconnection.

Piaget (1930) has shown how the child's grasp of causal relationships involves many inaccurate conceptions before the integration of experience and the development of maturity and intelligence bring him to an increasingly correct understanding of cause and effect: that the wind makes the trees move, and not that the movement of the trees creates the wind; that the word "sun" is a name created arbitrarily by people and not an intrinsic part of the bright disk in the daylight sky which came into their minds by gazing at the sun itself. The three year old who says "I can blow that apartment house over if I want to" is experimenting with ideas of cause and effect and his relation to them. The persistence of such thinking indicates the child's lack of mastery of his environment.

It is in helping to increase such mastery for the schizophrenic child that parent guidance may play a role. The child's need for repetition of action and speech can be met by doing things over and over again in the learning process. Because of his greater comfort with objects and with their laws of behavior, we can select objects to focus on first. If we provide a repetitious and familiar background, we can begin to introduce a pattern for change that can be used to meet other changes.

For example, if a schizophrenic child had a marked affective deviation, we would advise the parents to train him in a series of acceptable behaviors, so that his actions would resemble normal affective behavior. The schizophrenic child can learn by rote a portion of what the normal child learns intuitively. While his acquired behavior will not restore him to normal functioning, it will make it possible for him to respond more appropriately to his environment. He can learn that if he hits another child it is likely that he will get a blow in return. He can also learn that if he knocks over an object, he will meet less aggressive retaliation if he expresses regret and offers to help repair the damage.

Another prominent symptom of schizophrenic children is a tendency toward narrow, compulsive interests. As long as the child's interests are not dangerous or disruptive, we would advise parents and educators to let him continue with his idiosyncracies. In some cases, these interests may be channeled with positive results. For example, if the child has a compulsive preoccupation with moving parts of toys, this could in time be developed into a competent or even expert knowledge of engines. His obsessiveness may be directed by the parents into an interest in learning the routines of social amenity. If the child is bright, he may ultimately become involved in formal learning situations in which his peculiarities will be tolerated. However, if the schizophrenic child's obsessions lead to bizarre or possibly dangerous behavior, a definite and concerted effort must be made to remove them from his repertoire.

Of course, treatment and guidance methods must be individualized according to the severity of pathology, the amount of responsiveness manifested by the child and the ability of the parents to cooperate. For instance, with an autistic child whose awareness of the environment is minimal, handling must first be organized so as to elicit some indication of the youngster's ability to respond. The parents must announce an event and then have it happen, and this must be done again and again to see if the child can grasp any idea of linkage between the two occurrences. Only if he displays some responsiveness should one try to go further. Putting the child in a nursery school class may then be effective in giving him some idea of normative behavior. Perhaps the use of a teaching machine will help his formal education by giving him the endless repetition he needs without the impatience a human teacher might show.

Some of these procedures were used with Gene, an autistic child. His parents were given guidance, and they used considerable initiative in putting the therapist's suggestions into practice. For example, they searched for and found an excellent nursery school that agreed to admit the child. At home, they provided him with prime examples of "model" or normal behavior. In addition, a younger, nonschizophrenic brother was a great ally in that he gave Gene an opportunity to feel important.

The mother tried to get Gene to take notice of his brother, encouraging him to play with him and take care of the younger child. In Gene's presence, she repeatedly warned the toddler to stay on the sidewalk and keep out of the street. One day, when the mother had temporarily gone out of sight while the two children were outside, the younger boy wandered into the street. Gene became extremely agitated and ran to his mother, telling her that the baby was in the street and might get hurt. This, of course, was a great step forward in bringing the boy out of his autistic withdrawal, demonstrating his ability to react with correct affect to his family environment.

In other cases, the presence of a younger sibling may be helpful in giving the schizophrenic child someone at his own behavioral level with whom to communicate.

Sometimes hypermotility rather than obsessions or autism is chiefly responsible for interfering with a schizophrenic child's awareness of his environment. In such cases, it may be appropriate to use medications to decrease the activity level. Only after the child has been quieted down may it become possible for him to respond to environmental cues.

Direct treatment of the child may also be necessary at times to further the child's relatedness or improve his patterns of behavior.

Direct therapy is also appropriate for dealing with the acute fears a schizophrenic child may develop or for helping him through various periods of adjustment, such as a change in the family or physical environment.

For those children who have some awareness of the environment and of those who people it, a rehabilitative therapeutic approach may be the treatment of choice. In general, such an approach involves seven basic steps:

1. One small segment of reality, some object, is employed as a basis for activity.

2. The physical nature of this object is explored. It is compared with other objects and the laws governing its behavior under varying circumstances are examined.

3. In the course of play, these laws are stated and restated.

4. Differences between the object and the young patient are established in terms of the play activity being carried on.

5. New activities are introduced one by one, and as each enters the treatment situation, the pattern of stating the laws governing the activity is repeated. The play is structured so as to necessitate an examination and definition of what is being done.

6. People are brought into the discussion and the significance of human wishes and desires is explained in the same kind of terms that were applied to objects.

7. Rules of behavior are discussed and demonstrated. These include: what is expected of one in a given set of circumstances; what are good manners; what is meant by sharing; or, by contrast, what hurts others or makes them uncomfortable. If necessary, an issue is made of forbidding or of demanding certain forms of behavior.

This plan of treatment, based on principles of rehabilitation, represents an alternative to treatment directed toward the development of an affective relationship. Implicit in the treatment program described is acceptance of the concept of physiologic dysfunctioning of a still unknown nature as the basic disturbance and handicap which makes it difficult for the schizophrenic child to master his environment.

It is my belief that these children can best be aided, not by guarding them from tensions due to physiologic crisis, but by training them to meet special environmental demands so they will be better able to cope with subsequent crises of a similar nature. Periods of great change, such as adolescence, may bring with them not only turmoil and destructive strife but also unique possibilities for resolving conflicts and facing issues; new motivations and constructive strivings often appear at these times.

Changes in the environment are notoriously difficult for the schizophrenic youngster to master. Since life itself necessarily brings changes, however, any that he can be helped to master will provide him with a pattern and rules by which future changes can be more effectively tackled. Much of the aid may appear to be given mechanically and by rote, but it it nevertheless effective in terms of the handicapped child.

The therapist attempts to make the issues clear as early as possible in treatment. He lets the child know, in whatever terms are appropriate, that his behavior is deviant. The child must be taught alternative, acceptable modes of behavior. Both parent guidance and direct treatment are means to this end.

Prognosis

Childhood schizophrenia is a chronic syndrome for which we do not as yet have a cure. The degree of pathology will affect prognosis. For example, the group of children identified as schizophrenic by Potter in the 1930's are probably to be classified as having severe pathology. In a follow-up study of these patients after thirty years, it was found that all but one had to be institutionalized (Bennett and Klein, 1966). The original diagnoses remained unchanged in most cases. In another follow-up study of eighty autistic children, Leon Eisenberg (1956) reports that about one-third of the patients made some degree of adequate social adjustment, one-third remained poorly adjusted but could continue in the community, and one-third had to be more or less permanently institutionalized.

Eisenberg and Kanner (1956) have suggested that an autistic child who has failed to develop language by the age of five years

has a poor prognosis. It is among those who have some meaningful
speech by this age that the best prognoses are to be found, although
a favorable outcome is by no means assured. Follow-up studies
by both Kanner and Eisenberg indicate that individual psychotherapy has neither helped nor hindered the schizophrenic child.
My own view is that there is more promise in parent guidance,
environmental manipulation and selective use of individual psychotherapy.

Manic-Depressive Psychosis

Manic-depressive psychosis occurs in adolescents, and presents
the same picture as in adults. The patient's mood will exhibit
marked changes, ranging from hopelessness to elation. In the
depressed state, which may last for days, weeks or months, the
patient may show loss of appetite, a tendency to sleep excessively
and an inability to perform his daily routine. During the phase of
elevated mood, he may have little need for sleep and may be bursting with energy and ideas.

In the preadolescent child, the existence of manic-depressive
psychosis is questionable. Some psychiatrists report that infants
and young children may have periodic depressions that are to be
considered as examples of manic-depressive psychosis. However,
depressions in the earlier age group usually can be traced to specific traumatic situations and are not cyclical. The hyperactivity
manifested by children is generally not considered the dynamic
equivalent of the adult manic phase.

Other Psychosis

Childhood psychosis may be caused by both acute and chronic
diseases that affect brain function. Any acute illness in which there
is extreme toxicity, hypertension or high temperature may be
involved, including such common conditions as tonsilitis or measles.
Sydenham's chorea and encephalitis in its inflammatory stage are
other examples of acute illnesses that act directly on the brain and
may cause temporary psychotic episodes. Severe toxic states resulting from carbon monoxide poisoning, blood poisoning and burns

may also cause transient psychotic reactions. A nephritis with symptomatic hypertension has been known to be the cause of temporary hallucinations that disappeared with a decrease in blood pressure.

The chronic diseases that can cause psychosis include congenital anomalies of the brain, degenerative diseases of the central nervous system, brain tumors and some inflammatory diseases of the brain. The possibility of organic disease should therefore be considered in all cases of delusions or hallucinations in young children.

A psychotic state that is caused by, or is secondary to, a systemic disease will follow the course of the disease. If the psychotic state is caused by a short-term disorder from which there is a complete recovery, it will take the form of an acute self-limited delirium. A psychosis caused by a progressive degenerative disease or neoplasm will either consistently increase in severity or have exacerbations and remissions, according to the course of the underlying pathology. In such cases, treatment of the psychosis consists of treatment of the basic illness, although a palliative approach to symptoms is always in order in medical practice.

SELECTED REFERENCES

Bender, L.: Childhood schizophrenia: a review. *Int. J. Psychiat.* 5:211-236, 1968.

Bennett, S., and Klein, H.: Childhood schizophrenia: 30 years later. *Amer. J. Psychiat.* 122:1121-1124, 1966.

Bleuler, E.: *Dementia Praecox or the Group of Schizophrenias.* New York, International Universities Press, 1950.

Bradley, C.: *Schizophrenia in Children.* New York, Macmillan, 1941.

Creak, M.: Childhood psychosis: a review of 100 cases. *Brit. J. Psychiat.* 109:84-89, 1963.

Eisenberg, L.: The autistic child in adolescence. *Amer. J. Psychiat.* 112:607-612, 1956.

Eisenberg, L., and Kanner, L.: Early infantile autism. *Amer. J. Orthopsychiat.* 26:556-566, 1956.

Friedhoff, A. J.: Metabolism of dimethoxyphenethylamine and its possible relationship to schizophrenia. *In* Romano, J. (Ed.): *The Origins of Schizophrenia.* Amsterdam, Excerpta Medica Foundation, 1967.

Goldfarb, W.: *Childhood Schizophrenia.* Cambridge, Harvard University Press, 1961.

Kallman, F. J., and Roth, B.: Genetic aspects of preadolescent schizophrenia. *Amer. J. Psychiat.* 112:599-606, 1956.

Kanner, L.: Problems of nosology and psychodynamics of early infantile autism. *Amer. J. Orthopsychiat.* 19:416-426, 1949.

Kanner, L.: *Child Psychiatry*. Springfield, Ill., Charles C Thomas, 1957.

Kety, S. S.: Biochemical theories of schizophrenia. *Science* 129:1528-1532, 1590-1596, 1959.

Mahler, M.: On child psychosis and schizophrenia: autistic and symbiotic infantile psychosis. *Psychoanal. Stud. Child* 7:286-305, 1952.

Maudsley, H.: *Physiology and Pathology of the Mind*. New York, D. Appleton, 1867.

Piaget, J.: *Child's Conception of Physical Causality*. New York, Harcourt, Brace, 1930.

Potter, H. W.: Schizophrenia in children. *Amer. J. Psychiat.* 12:1253-1270, 1933.

Rutter, M.: The influence of organic and emotional factors on the origins, nature, and outcome of child psychosis. *Develop. Med. Child Neurol.* 7:518, 1965.

de Sanctis, S.: *Neuropsichiatria Infantile*. Rome, Stock, 1925.

Wing, J. K. (Ed.): *Early Childhood Autism*. Oxford, Pergamon Press, 1966.

Wolff, S., and Chess, S.: A behavioral study of schizophrenic children. *Acta Psychiat. Scand.* 40:438-466, 1964.

Wolff, S., and Chess, S.: An analysis of the language of fourteen schizophrenic children. *J. Child Psychol. Psychiat.* 6:29-41, 1965.

13. Specific Learning Disabilities

DIFFICULTIES IN LEARNING are often associated with behavioral disturbances in children of school age. School is obviously a major influence in a child's life. In addition to its formal educational function, the classroom is the basis of the youngster's most important peer relationships. A learning problem may therefore engender feelings of inadequacy and shame that provoke various kinds of defensive behavior.

In diagnosing learning difficulties, it is essential to distinguish between (1) an emotional learning block in which the psychologic problem is primary and the defect is symptomatic, and (2) a specific disability caused by faulty neurologic function that directly interferes with the learning process and may lead secondarily to emotional disorder. Specific learning disabilities are also to be distinguished from general retardation of mental functioning, discussed in chapter 9. Mentally retarded children may have specific disabilities, but these are subordinate to the intellectual slowness as a whole.

In the past, the emotional aspects of learning problems were emphasized to the neglect of the neurologic factors. The tendency was to assume that a psychologic block accounted for the learning disorders of most children who came to psychiatric notice. Recently, however, it has been shown that many of these learning disabilities are organismic in origin.

A variety of reading, writing and speech disturbances, not associated with generalized mental defects, are found in children with a wide range of intellectual capacity. Some of these are related to maturational lags; as the child develops, the disability gradually disappears. Other impairments are permanent. Recognition of the primary nature of these disabilities has made it possible to elaborate therapeutic measures, including remedial learning and efforts to develop substitute mental pathways. As a result, an increasing proportion of children with learning difficulties are able to receive the special help they need rather than endless hours of inappropriate play therapy.

175

Language Disorders

The initial impetus to the study of language disturbances in childhood was given by Orton (1937). Pointing out that in normal development one hemisphere of the brain assumes dominance, he noted that "the establishment of the physiological habits of initiating the more intricate motor responses, such as speech and writing, from the association area of one hemisphere alone usually occurs early in childhood but at varying ages, and expresses itself outwardly in a preference for the right or left hand." Orton suggested that delays and defects in language development arise from either a failure to establish hemispheric dominance or external interference with the expression of dominance in the child's preferred hand. The latter point was especially pertinent during the era when teachers and parents insisted that left-handed children become right-handed.

Although some of Orton's original formulations now need to be modified, they opened up an important avenue of study. It has been found that the speech centers of many left-handed persons are located in the left hemisphere or have a bilateral representation, whereas right-handed children have unilateral representation in the contralateral hemisphere. With bilateral representation, the development of speech and written language may be slower and more vulnerable to interference. However, a more important index of whether a child's language disability is organic rather than motivational is right-left directional confusion, which does not always correlate absolutely with mixed cerebral dominance.

The most common of the developmental language disabilities is dyslexia, or difficulty in reading and writing. Dyslexic children manifest right-left disorientation. This shows up in the confusion of letters in the alphabet that are mirror images of each other, such as *d* and *b,* or *p* and *q.* There may also be a mixing up of letters that are mirrors of each other on another plane, such as *m* and *w.* In addition, whole words may be reversed, such as *was* and *saw,* or *dog* and *god.* This difficulty has been termed strephosymbolia (twisted symbols).

In the effort to perform well, dyslexic children may recognize a word or a group of words and then incorrectly read other words that contain the same letter groups. The problem may be obscured in a bright and conscientious child who will compensate for dyslexia to some extent by specially attentive listening. The gap between auditory and visual comprehension may be striking, and the child may be incorrectly criticized for being "sloppy" in his written productions. Spelling is notoriously poor, but scrutiny of the misspelled words often reveals an attempt to use phonetic clues.

If the problem is not identified at the outset, a host of defensive maneuvers may be set up which become more noticeable than the difficulty itself. The child may start to lie about whether he has homework at all, or he may copy some other children's written assignments. Many studies indicate that even with apparent compensation, due to both maturation and special training, spelling disabilities persist. In some cases a significant defect remains, and a child may need to have someone read to him if he is to be educated to intellectual capacity.

In problems connected with the development of spoken language, expressive aphasia is more common than receptive aphasia. Children with speech difficulties have an apparently normal comprehension of language, and their general adaptive development is not retarded. But their first word may not be spoken until they are three years old, perhaps even as late as five years. When the words do appear, they are often poorly enunciated, though the grammatical structure may be adequate. Sometimes the grammatical usage is so advanced that one suspects the child has actually been speaking for a longer time than his hearers have been able to recognize.

Some children with speech disability have such easy adaptability and cheerfulness that they can communicate with children by other means and be accepted as companions. But in most cases the behavioral reactions to such a disability are a significant part of the total presenting picture. Sensitive to the mockery they have experienced, some children refuse to talk at all except with a chosen few with whom they are comfortable. They may give an appearance of mutism. They may seem extremely shy or very aggressive. It is not always easy to judge whether these behavioral manifestations are reactions to their negative experiences or are independent problems.

Receptive aphasia is most difficult to diagnose with assurance. A developmental aphasia that affects comprehension is such a fundamental disability that it must interfere with the development of normal processes and relationships. As a result, it is difficult to distinguish between a primary thinking disorder, in which the language aberration is merely symptomatic, and a primary speech disorder, in which failure of communication causes the child to get distorted messages from the environment.

It is also difficult to distinguish between aphasia and a language dysfunction that is symptomatic of a generalized organic cerebral disorder, mental defect or infantile autism. The problem of differentiation is compounded if there is a disturbance in behavior that is either secondary to the language disability or unrelated etiologically. The diagnosis of aphasia is made only when there is an indication that the child is capable of ideation well above his speech level.

For example, a mute child of six who uses toys at a level appropriate for his age and whose history indicates activities commensurate with chronologic age may be diagnosed as aphasic. On the other hand, a mute six year old who merely piles up blocks, who cannot play with toy furniture and human figure dolls in a functional way, and whose history indicates no activities above what would be expected of an infant of eighteen months, would not be diagnosed as aphasic. Such a child's speech retardation is one manifestation of a general slowness in mentation.

A further diagnostic differentiation must be made between aphasia and the retarded or distorted use of language found in infantile autism. In the latter category, the primary disturbance is considered to be lack of interest in the environment, not lack of capacity for mentation.

Other Learning Disabilities

While language disorders have been more thoroughly studied than other problems, certain nonverbal factors are beginning to be investigated as sources of learning difficulties.

There may be a lag or unevenness in the ability to integrate two sensory functions or a sensory and a motor function. Thus, auditory-visual, visual-haptic or visual-motor correlations may be faulty. This phenomenon has been studied by Birch (1964) and others. As a first step, developmental norms for these integrative capacities are being identified.

The child who has difficulty in integrating sensory clues may be gaining no benefit from traditional methods of instruction. In spelling drill, for example, a teacher customarily asks the child to look at a word, say it, and then write it. If the child cannot match visual and auditory stimuli, such drill becomes an obstacle to learning instead of a reinforcement.

Similarly, some children have difficulty in their perceptual-motor competence: they cannot reproduce a visual perception. Obviously, careful testing is required to determine if the difficulty lies in the realm of perception or motor ability.

Other "input" handicaps include color blindness, inability to make figure-background distinctions, partial deafness, and a central deafness in which the child hears all the tones but is unable to give them symbolic meaning. These defects must also be kept in mind as possible sources of specific learning disabilities.

The psychiatrist should inquire into several other learning factors. Can the child conceptualize appropriately? Do attentional difficulties prevent his hearing more than a fraction of what is told to him? Does he have difficulty in retaining what he has learned because of deficiencies in memory?

While the child psychiatrist is not expected to be a specialist in the administration of tests to identify learning disabilities, he must be aware of these defects and the methods for assessing and correcting them. He should have some competence in screening, so he can recognize the signs of a learning disability requiring a battery of tests to determine its nature and severity.

Hereditary Factors

In some cases there is a clear family history of specific learning disability. When a youngster presents with serious school problems, the possibility of a genetic pattern should be investigated. If a familial history of late language development can be identified, it suggests that the child patient may not be retarded. This provides some basis for reassuring the parents that the child will eventually use language normally.

Language disabilities are found more often in boys than in girls. The data indicate that these disabilities may follow the pattern of a recessive hereditary characteristic.

Treatment

The appropriate treatment of a specific learning disability is determined by the total evaluation of the child. If the situation is recognized very early, before the child has become demoralized, it may be possible to meet his needs with remedial work tailored to his disability.

The timing of remedial measures depends on the maturation of brain function. Premature remediation will do no good; indeed it has the negative effect of reinforcing the child's sense of discouragement. At the appropriate time, remedial measures should deal with both the learning disability and the emotional block the child may have developed.

If the specific dysfunction is permanent, as in word blindness, a different strategy is necessary. After remedial efforts have been exhausted and retesting has confirmed the basic organic difficulty, teaching efforts are addressed to training the child for compensatory development of his intact capacities.

If the child has developed secondary emotional problems, these must be taken into account in determining the appropriate treatment methods. Emotional disturbances may occur because the youngster with a sensory or motor speech difficulty has been cut off from communication with his peers during the time when a child normally begins to learn to exchange ideas with other children, to play cooperatively and to assert himself with them. A child who lacks adequate speech is rejected by other children; he is thrown into a prolonged dependency relationship with adults, which may be the nucleus of a dependency-hostility relationship with his parents and sibs.

Sometimes a child with learning disabilities has become so discouraged that he actually functions as the retardate he has been taken to be. Or he may develop a host of defensive maneuvers, such as clowning, which give him a spurious sense of mastery. In some cases, the emotional problems must be dealt with before the child will be able to accept remedial work. In other instances, it is advisable to give the child remedial work first and then, when a plateau is reached, to reevaluate his emotional state. Medication, direct psychotherapy or parent guidance may be the initial treatment approach called for in a given case.

Parent guidance is an important form of therapy when a child with a specific learning disability develops secondary emotional problems. Unfortunately, it is all too easy to assume that the parents are responsible for the child's behavior and lack of learning. When a teacher reports to the parents that the child daydreams or pays no attention in class, they address themselves to these "problems"; they are not oriented toward investigating possible organismic defects and assume that the expert's report is valid. As a result, they may restrict the child's activities so that he will study more or punish him for bringing home reports of his bad behavior. They are not necessarily pressuring individuals and, on the contrary, may conceivably be trying to carry out what they've been told to do. However, their behavior may be contributing to a noxious parent-child interaction and further demoralizing the child or exacerbating his difficulties, the opposite of what the parents are trying to do. Parent guidance may therefore be a crucial component of therapy.

Emotional Learning Block

If the learning difficulty is diagnosed as an emotional block, therapeutic efforts are directed toward overcoming the emotional problem. Once this has been done, remedial academic assistance is usually required to enable the child to fill in the gaps in his knowledge and learn the techniques he has missed while suffering from the block.

To give effective treatment to such a child, the therapist must ascertain the nature of the block and when in the child's development it arose. The implication here is that the child's emotional difficulties antedated the formal learning situation, and that they were of such a nature as to impede his potential ability to acquire knowledge. Such a situation may arise when a parent is impelled by prestige needs to demand high educational achievement, and at the same time the child has an attitude of hostility and negativism toward the parent. The child identifies learning as a gift to the demanding parent which his negativism makes him withhold. As a result, he is unable to respond to teaching. An emotional block may also arise when a child associates learning with growing up and with being forced to abandon his dependency, or when he is apprehensive about the authority of the teacher and manifests his fears by intellectual paralysis.

As a result of these and other neurotic mechanisms, a child may be unable to respond to teaching—unable to learn—despite the fact that under other emotional circumstances he would have adequate mental capacity to master the subject matter. If this is the case, one should arrange for individual tutoring concurrent with psychotherapy.

SELECTED REFERENCES

Birch, H. (Ed.): *Brain Damage in Children*. Baltimore, Williams & Wilkins, 1964.

Critchley, M.: *Developmental Dyslexia*. Springfield, Ill., Charles C Thomas, 1964.

de Hirsch, K., Jansky, J. J., and Langford, W. S.: *Predicting Reading Failure*. New York, Harper & Row, 1966.

Johnson, D. J., and Myklebust, H. R.: *Learning Disabilities*. New York, Grune & Stratton, 1967.

Money, J. (Ed.): *Reading Disability: Progress and Research Needs in Dyslexia*. Baltimore, Johns Hopkins Press, 1962.

Morley, M. E.: *The Development and Disorders of Speech*. Baltimore, Williams & Wilkins, 1965.

Myklebust, H. R. (Ed.): *Progress in Learning Disabilities*. New York, Grune & Stratton, 1967.

O'Connor, N., and Hermelin, B.: *Speech and Thought in Severe Subnormality*. New York, Macmillan, 1963.

Orton, S.: *Reading, Writing and Speech Problems in Children*. New York, W. W. Norton, 1937.

Vygotsky, L. S.: *Thought and Language*. Cambridge, MIT Press, 1962.

14. Problems Arising from Special Stress Situations

A NUMBER of special stress situations in childhood may give rise to problems that must be dealt with as expeditiously as possible. Among the circumstances that can produce stress are physical illnesses and handicaps, hospitalization, separation, adoption and issues connected with a child's socioeconomic and cultural identification.

Physical Illness and Handicaps

Psychologic stress in childhood is often associated with a physical illness or handicap present at birth or having its onset in the early years. The physical defect may affect the child's subsequent personality development. Restrictions on activity and social life may provide fertile soil for the development of psychiatric disorders. In this regard, sensitive pediatric handling can play a preventive role in minimizing or eliminating destructive behavioral adaptations.

The problem of adaptation to a physical illness or handicap differs according to whether it is present at birth or appears later. The youngster who has had a motility disturbance from birth is not aware during his early development that his abilities fall short of the normal. A different kind of adjustment must be made by the child who has learned to walk, climb and skip, and then loses these abilities through accident or disease. Similarly, the psychologic issues involved in the dietary handling of celiac disease or multiple allergies to food differ according to whether they arise before the child is old enough to digest a full diet or after he has learned to enjoy foods which must now be denied him. Still other psychologic issues are involved in rheumatic fever with a permanent cardiac disability and in a recurrent asthmatic condition with periodic disability, or in partial blindness and deafness.

In all these situations, irrespective of the degree and quality of disability or the time of onset of the disease, some children have a healthy, constructive development and others have an unhealthy and distorted one. Some children accept their limitations realistically and involve themselves in activities and interpersonal relationships to the full extent of their capacity. Others deny the presence of the handicap or greatly magnify it; they may be fearful of all new situations, avoid interpersonal relationships and develop phobias and compulsions. In short, the nature of the illness, its extent and the timing of its onset do not automatically signal success or failure of adaptation.

The concept of mastery is useful in clarifying the issues of psychologic stress that must be faced by children with physical illnesses and handicaps. The child is enabled to achieve mastery of his handicap by being taught the nature of its manifestations and effective ways of functioning within its framework. This definition of the illness must, of course, be comprehensible to the child at his specific age, and it has to be presented in terms that relate to his everyday functioning. For example, the three year old with a food allergy can be made to understand that oranges, lemons and grapefruit give him the rash which he dislikes, and he can learn that when someone offers him one of these fruits he must refuse if he wishes to avoid discomfort. The diabetic child who is invited to a birthday party can learn that he may eat a few goodies at the party only if he has restricted his usual diet, according to plan, earlier in the day. The child with a cardiac defect is capable of learning that he may participate in sports only if he can be relied upon to withdraw from a game at the first signs of fatigue.

A child's mastery of his illness also involves his learning how and when remedial medical measures are to be taken. The asthmatic child can learn that he is to take a specific medicine at the first croupy cough or the first sign of wheezing in order to avoid or minimize a severe asthmatic attack. A young asthmatic child can be made responsible for announcing the early stages of an attack; an older child with adequate coordination can assume responsibility for taking the proper medication himself.

The youngster with a physical handicap who knows what he can do without help and what activities legitimately call for outside aid is moving toward self-sufficiency. He is less likely to be afraid of new situations than the youngster who has been allowed to become overdependent or who is ashamed to ask for aid. In short, the child who is adjusting well to his illness limits the handicap to its actual physical manifestations.

But a child who has an obvious physical disability is psychologically vulnerable because of his difficulty in keeping up with his peers in various activities, because of parent-child differences in how to handle the handicap, or for a host of other reasons. With appropriate handling, the child's vulnerability need not be converted into neurotic behavior. Often, however, the child who has adjusted poorly to his illness extends the handicap beyond its physical manifestations. His behavior may come to show overdependence, bravado, refusal to accept proffered aid, obsequiousness, sensitivity to criticism or a variety of other neurotic attitudes. As a result, the child now has the added handicap of maladaptive behavior, and this may influence his interpersonal relationships even more than his physical defect. He may come to feel that others dislike him because of his illness, when actually they are reacting to his behavior.

The child's psychologic response to his illness may sometimes intensify his organic condition. For example, if a diabetic child reacts to his disease with denial and fails to take his medicine or stick to his diet, he may develop severe complications. Similarly, if a child ignores the restrictions that may relieve his allergic manifestations, he may develop chronic effects of eczema. The exacerbated medical problems may require that the child be kept out of school for long periods of time, with an adverse effect on both peer relations and scholastic achievement.

Parents, too, play a role in determining the psychiatric consequences of illness and the special stresses on the child. In many cases, they overestimate the amount of restriction and care that must be given. If the child has been permitted to exploit his illness in order to gain extra attention and special privileges, he may develop a vested interest in maintaining the privileged position of being ill. On the other hand, if the parents are not realistic about the handicap and get annoyed with the child in situations that call for patience and help, he is unlikely to learn to handle these situations in a healthy manner. There are even parents who threaten to withhold medication as a disciplinary measure, with the child in turn using refusal of medication as a retaliatory weapon.

Pediatric awareness of such issues is essential. If the physician who takes care of the child fails to discuss the nature of the illness or handicap adequately with the parents, there is likely to be inappropriate management. Later, after the child has developed a well-defined behavioral problem, psychiatric investigation may reveal that his hostility-dependency pattern, fanciful tale-telling or inability to have an organized approach to learning gained its initial impetus from poor parental handling of a congenitally dislocated hip, hypertrophic pyloric stenosis or outgrown baby croup. An understanding of the genesis of the behavior pattern is a potent weapon in reversing it.

Consideration of the proper psychologic handling of a child's illness should start when it is first diagnosed. Here it is important to differentiate between the child who is bedridden with an acute and self-limited disease, and the youngster whose illness is long-term or chronic. Hospitalization raises specific additional issues.

Acute Illness

With acute illness, a child is entitled to an extra amount of diversion and attention, in addition to whatever medical procedure is required. Certain illnesses may call for reassurance, if the child is frightened. For example, the youngster with considerable pain or with a delirium caused by high fever may be rather frightened about the meaning of his symptoms. In such situations, it is essential that the child be reassured and that his extra needs be satisfied.

After such an illness, many children attempt to maintain the interpersonal relationship that yielded special privileges. The parent's responsibility is to restore the relationship that existed prior to the illness. It should be made clear to the child that continued exploitation of the dependency situation is not possible. Often the child is actually reassured by the refusal to give him extra attention, since it indicates that he has really recovered.

A problem of dependency behavior initiated by an illness requires careful study and treatment. It may be necessary to analyze the basic parent-child relationship, as well as the actual events of the illness. The child may have been given an inadequate explanation of his illness, and may have anxieties that he cannot bring himself to express for fear of being ridiculed. In other situations, there may have been an antecedent behavioral difficulty which was sharpened and clarified by the events of the illness. It may then be possible for the parent gradually to modify the child's dependency feeling by carefully evaluating each situation and demanding that the child carry through what he is clearly capable of doing successfully. If such measures do not bring about the desired results, a psychologic diagnostic investigation may be required.

Chronic Illness

When the acute phase of an illness is over and it is clear that the disabling condition will be chronic or intermittent, or that there is a permanent physical handicap, the manner in which the child is handled thereafter may determine his attitude toward true mastery of his physical state. The scale may be tipped in the direction of his dominating the situation by his helplessness and dependency, or he may be started in the direction of realizing that the more independent he is the more rewarding life will be for him.

Throughout all of these situations, it is important to bear in mind that the child's medical needs always take priority over his psychologic needs. Although necessary medical procedures should always be carried out in as palatable and acceptable a way as possible, the decision to give the child a certain medication is determined by his illness and not by his psychologic reactions. In general, one will obtain better cooperation from a child who understands why certain procedures are being introduced, is given warning when they are planned and is informed when they will hurt. These explanations, however, are given to obtain the child's cooperation, not his permission. When a youngster objects to medical procedures either through panic or negativism, they should be carried out as quickly as possible in order to cut short the period of commotion.

Hospitalization

Hospitalization is indicated for the physically ill child who requires surgical procedures or a medical-nursing regime available only in specialized institutional settings. More and more hospitals are accommodating semiprivate patients in pediatric wards instead of small rooms. The more pleasant and cheerful the atmosphere of a children's ward, the easier will be the adjustment of the sick child. In general, he is more contented in a hospital if he is with other children than if he is shut up in a room alone. This, of course, does not apply to the extremely ill child who is in no condition to be aware of or interested in the company of others.

The child who enters the hospital for an operation may come for an emergency procedure, such as an appendectomy, or for elective surgery. Where the situation is acute and critical, there is little time to prepare the child. It is only necessary for the parent to tell him that an operation is to take place and to give him as much explanation of the hospital routine as is possible under the circumstances. Elective procedures include tonsillectomy, eye operations, herniorrhaphies and cosmetic operations. If one of these is to be performed, it is necessary to explain to the child, in terms appropriate to his age and understanding, what the operation will consist of from his point of view. For example, if he is to come into the hospital in the morning, have a blood count, a preanesthetic injection, and then go to sleep, it is necessary merely to describe these procedures. The stretcher ride to the operating room need not be described. If, however, the child is to be operated on under local anesthesia, the preparation should include the details of the stretcher ride to the operating room and what he will be asked to do to cooperate. A child who has not been adequately informed about this procedure may misunderstand, even to the point of believing that he is going to his death. The after-effects of the operation should also be explained to the child in terms that will have meaning for him——where it will hurt, whether his eyes will be bandaged, what activity restrictions there will be, what foods he may and may not have, and so on.

Children who become tearful, fearful and sleepless when hospitalized are displaying separation anxiety. This, however, involves more than the fact that the child is away from his mother, as might be the case if he were visiting a relative or traveling with his grandparents. What also must be considered is the fact that the child is in a new environment: the room is set up strangely, the noises and smells are unfamiliar, there is a new group of youngsters with whom he has to interact, and the nurses not only differ physically from his mother but also play a different role and are not there to amuse him. One must be aware of all these new stimuli and the demands for adaptation they imply, and not limit consideration to the fact of separation from the mother alone. Furthermore, the child's reaction is likely to be colored by his temperamental characteristics. The youngster who is highly adaptable may warm up quickly and have a grand old time in the hospital. By contrast, the child who adapts slowly in other situations is likely to be slow to warm up here, too, and this must be handled for what it is, and not necessarily as part of separation anxiety.

Separation Anxiety

The term separation anxiety implies that, whatever the situation, removal of a child from his mother specifically causes anxiety. I believe that the term is often used too loosely. While some children react with anxiety to any separation, others show a differentiated response depending on the situation.

Different children will have had varying experiences before they first face a real separation from their mother and the need to relate to other persons. Thus, for some youngsters, attendance at nursery school or kindergarten is neither the first such separation nor is it the first structured group experience. Some children may have spent periods of time with relatives or other adults, away from home, and some may have had preschool play-group experiences. For the former, the structured demands of school will be new and possibly stressful, whereas for the latter, separation from the mother is the new demand to master. Other children may arrive at school having had no experience either away from their parents or in a group situation, and for them the experience will be most stressful.

How the child adapts to these demands will depend in great part on his temperamental characteristics. A child who readily approaches new situations and adapts quickly to them is unlikely to display anxiety at separation from his mother. On the other hand, the child who is slow to warm up is likely to show such anxiety if he is asked to adapt to all the new demands quickly and at one time. How one handles the child to avoid maladaptation, therefore, depends on his characteristic pattern of reactivity. The first child may sail right into the classroom without a backward glance at his mother. In fact, he may be annoyed if she stays around. The shy child needs a more gradual process of acclimatization. First he must get used to the physical set-up of the room while his mother keeps him company. Then, he can become attached to a teacher, though his mother remains present. Eventually, he spends a longer and longer period of time in school without his parent, until finally she need not come at all. Throughout this process, one gives the child a chance to make his connection with a new object or person by using something familiar as the bridge. Such tactics may be necessary in other situations too, but at all times they must be applied only in response to the child's specific personality needs.

Socioeconomic and Cultural Stresses

Special circumstances associated with a child's socioeconomic and cultural identification may be sources of stress to him. More and more attention is being paid to the special vulnerabilities of children from slum and ghetto areas. These children are likely to have more physical illness and disability than the children of families with more money. Their prenatal care is less favorable. They are more likely to have had suboptimal diet in their early years, to have ingested noxious substances, to have sustained accidental injuries. All of these experiences may contribute to behavior disorders.

In addition there is a dissonance between some of the cultural patterns the child learns in adapting to the mores of his family and those of the larger society in which he must learn, work and live. Such dissonance can constitute a stress, even though there is nothing intrinsically inferior or superior in the culture of the child's background.

The special stresses upon lower-class children are particularly evident in their formal learning experiences. First of all, they are usually not oriented in their early years toward task completion or intellectual exercises such as those provided by "educational toys." Unlike middle-class parents, those of lower-class children often do not assume responsibility for preparing the child for education: they have the quite reasonable attitude that it is the school's job to teach the child. As a result, the children enter school less prepared to be taught by teachers who come largely from the middle class and are geared to youngsters with their own kind of background. The teacher, using a middle-class standard or model of what to expect, frequently responds to the lower-class child's approach to school with annoyance because he is not addressing himself to the work but is being "naughty" or "inattentive." This further adds to the stresses on the lower-class child. If he tries to be good and behaves as he has been taught to be good—being quiet and nonresponsive and not interfering—the teachers frequently assume he is not interested or else is stupid. The teacher's negative response to his attempts to behave further bewilder him. Stress accumulates, and an unhealthy interaction between teacher and child becomes likely.

Lower-class children are often referred for psychiatric treatment because of teacher complaints that they are inattentive, disruptive or in a world of their own. Specifically, teachers may request information about the child's intellectual ability since he doesn't catch on to instruction or looks frightened and never answers in class. Obviously, these may be symptoms of retardation or of significant psychiatric disorders. However, the psychiatrist must be alert to the possibility that this also may be a reactive behavior problem due to a clash between the teacher's and child's styles. The lower-class youngster comes to school ready to learn, but not in terms of the structure that fits the middle-class child and teacher. Awareness of this will keep the psychiatrist from making an incorrect diagnosis and recommending inappropriate therapy.

Lower-class children are faced with other stresses in their school years. Schools in the slums often have inexperienced teachers, and there are frequent changes of teaching personnel. As the child progresses from grade to grade, his learning deficits pile up. Thus, children with intellectual capacities that would otherwise permit them to learn may develop defeatist attitudes and reactive behavior disorders. They do not acquire skills that will permit them to have a higher education or expanded vocational opportunities. This becomes a stressful experience, and not uncommonly the child becomes demoralized with regard to his being able to determine what his future will be—"What's the use?" In such circumstances, dropping out of school and delinquency are understandable adaptations. In turn, the youngster's parents attack him for his behavior, thus adding to the demands on him; or they rise to his defense uncritically, thus reinforcing the child's belligerent attitude to school and making the situation even harder to resolve.

The psychiatrist, in forming his evaluation, must take this socioeconomically derived stress into full account. With such awareness, he can more accurately assess the specific nature of each child's behavior disorder. He is enabled to differentiate between poor learning exposure, specific learning disabilities and cerebral dysfunction. In short, he can distinguish between the child's ability to learn and his current competence.

One must also consider the ethnic background of the child in investigating the specific stresses he faces. The psychiatrist must familiarize himself with the cultural mores, especially the child-care practices and attitudes toward task completion and interpersonal relationships, of the specific group to which a child belongs. Similarly, full recognition must be given to the consequences of discrimination faced by the Negro child or the youngster who comes from any other easily identified minority group.

In focusing on the negative effects of stress experienced by "disadvantaged" children, we should keep in mind that positive reaction to stress can also be strengthening. As Robert Coles (1967) has so vividly reported, children under extraordinary pressures can show great resourcefulness. They may also present a quite different picture of their adaptive capacities to a stranger than to a member of their own group.

Middle-class children, too, are faced with certain stresses characteristic of their group. For example, as a result of a high-income family's excessive emphasis on academic success as measured by good grades, a child may work toward pleasing the teacher and his parents rather than mastering the subject matter. A middle-class child of average intelligence may develop feelings of inferiority because he is in competition with classmates who have higher IQs, and even a child of superior intelligence may be under great stress if the family norm is above his capacity. Competitive striving becomes most intense in high school, when the pressure mounts to achieve grades for admission to colleges with prestige. Many children do not know what profession they want to follow, but feel a terrible necessity to declare themselves long before they have had a chance to explore various possibilities. Lower-class children do not usually face this special stress unless theirs is an upwardly mobile family.

Adoption

In general, the problems that arise between parents and adopted children are the same as those that would occur, given the same personalities and circumstances, if the children were not adopted. These problems, however, may be intensified in the adoptive situation. Thus, a mother who would in any case tend to be overprotective may be even more so with a child who has been adopted after many years of sterility or unsuccessful pregnancies. A naturally overindulgent father may be more indulgent with his adopted child who came into the family after years of planning and waiting.

If the child has been adopted in an attempt to hold a shaky marriage together, he is likely to be maladjusted; but this is also true of the child who was conceived for the same purpose. Mature persons whose marriage is stable are generally successful and conscientious parents, regardless of whether they achieve parenthood through conception or adoption. The biologic bond in itself has no magical power to tie people closely.

Many of the problems that appear to stem from adoption actually arise because adults tend to assume that what bothers them also bothers their children, that facts which have disturbing connotations for them have similar connotations for their children. A case in point is the concern often felt by today's adoptive mother about the effect on her child of learning that he did not grow in her body. The situation is ironic, in view of the fact that only a few generations ago such information was believed to be traumatic and was kept from children by telling them that the stork brought them, that they were found in cabbages, or carried into the house by the doctor in his little black bag. It is the adoptive mother who is disturbed by the fact that her child did not grow in her body, not the child.

To the child, facts have the connotations given to them by his life experience. Adoption will be shameful to a child only if the fact is treated by the parents as shameful, covered up, and finally admitted with reluctance.

It is a mistake to regard adoption in itself as a source of potential difficulty that must constantly be kept in mind. But it is also erroneous to assume that it is of no importance. The fact of adoption is of great significance for both parents and child. To the parents, its meaning should be defined, so that it is neither underestimated nor given undue importance. The child, too, needs to know the facts of his relationship to his family and how and why he became a member. His interests, ideas and confusions about this aspect of his life will change as he grows older, just as his interests, ideas and confusions about other aspects will change. If his questions about adoption are answered in a manner appropriate to his developmental needs, without overinsistence on problems or refusal to acknowledge their existence, he will be able to master this phase of his life as constructively as he masters others.

When the parent-child relationship is disturbed, parent and child alike tend to blame the difficulty on the fact that the child is adopted. But the adoption is usually a secondary and complicating factor, almost never the nucleus of the difficulty. It is important to keep in mind that types of behavior difficulties and parent-child conflict are the same, as noted above, in adoptive situations and in situations where the parent-child bond is biologic. The child who feels rejected, for example, may try to find a rational explanation for his feeling in the fact that he is adopted. Actually, he feels rejected because he is indeed being rejected or because he misinterprets parental actions and attitudes. In dealing with behavioral problems of adopted children, once the special meaning of the adoptive situation has been clarified, the diagnostic study and therapeutic planning should be carried out in the same way as in any other case.

SELECTED REFERENCES

Bowlby, J., Ainsworth, M., Boston, M., and Rosenbluth, D.: The effects of mother-child separation: A follow-up study. Brit. J. Med. Psychol. 29:211-247, 1956.

Coles, R.: Children of Crisis. Boston, Little, Brown & Co., 1967.

Carter, V., and Chess, S.: Factors influencing the adaptations of organically handicapped children. Amer. J. Orthopsychiat. 21:827-837, 1951.

Deutsch, F., and Nadell, R.: Psychosomatic aspects of dermatology with special consideration of allergic phenomena. Nervous Child. 5:339-364, 1946.

Festinger, L.: Cognitive dissonance. Sci. Amer. 207:93, Oct., 1962.

Freud, A.: The role of bodily illness in the mental life of children. Psychoanalytic Study of the Child, Vol. 7. New York, International Universities Press, 1952.

Yarrow, L. J.: Maternal deprivation: Toward an empirical and conceptual re-evaluation. Psychol. Bull. 58:459-490, 1961.

15. Adolescent Behavior Problems

MOST YOUNG PEOPLE PASS from childhood dependency to the semidependent status of adolescence without serious difficulty. This fact tends to be obscured by the public attention drawn to the behavior problems of adolescents who do not make the transition smoothly. Often overlooked, too, is the fact that a state of turmoil is not abnormal for a youngster at this stage of development. The physical changes of puberty, the social adjustments, and the need to make vocational and other decisions give rise to pressing problems.

A young person's ability to solve these "normal problems" depends in large part on the opportunities he has to discuss them freely with parents, trusted adult advisers, older siblings and friends. In some cases there is no outward evidence of turmoil; but where understanding and communication are poor, the classic signs may be noted in the frequent arguments between adolescent and parent about such issues as hair style and curfew arrangements.

In assessing adolescent behavioral problems, the therapist must take into account the special characteristics of this period of development, extending roughly from twelve to eighteen years of age. To begin with, it is important to recognize that individual physical differences play a particularly important role after puberty. Youngsters become intensely conscious of any physical deviation from the group, such as shortness of stature in a boy or underdeveloped secondary sex characteristics in a girl. The psychiatrist has to avoid giving undue weight to such factors, which may be only an incidental feature of an underlying pathology. At the same time, one must recognize that a youngster's physical deviations and his reaction to them may make him appear to be more disturbed than he is intrinsically.

Adolescents typically follow an erratic course between dependence and independence. It is a mistake to consider dependence and independence as mutually exclusive, one defining childhood and one defining adulthood. The adolescent swings between the two poles. Youngsters who are really finding their way to a healthy independence are also able to select those circumstances in which they are in fact dependent and must ask for help. If something arises that is truly beyond his ability to handle, the secure adolescent will turn to his parents for support. The therapist must differentiate between mature independence and mere bravado or an inappropriate insistence on the formality of independence when this is merely a desire to be unsupervised. Similarly, one must be careful not to equate situations in which an individual shows good judgment by turning to others for legitimate assistance and situations in which the adolescent leans on others for servicing that he can actually do himself or should at least be striving to master.

The behavioral problems of adolescents must also be understood and handled in terms of their special areas of expression. In both children and adolescents, behavior patterns and personality attributes are expressed in activities that may be constructive, neutral or destructive. Adolescents, however, by the very fact that they are nearly full grown physically and have greater mobility than children, have a wider range of activities and more diversified modes of expression. The young child is limited to his immediate neighborhood and school in seeking his peer group. His desires and conflicts are usually expressed within the pattern of one of the peer groups that is within easy reach. He may exercise some selectivity in aligning himself with one of several groups, but beyond this he has actually only the choice of fitting in or not belonging—that is, isolating himself from peer relationships. The adolescent, by contrast, can range further afield in seeking a peer group in which to express his behavioral attributes. Thus the competitive teenager with a drive for dangerous and perhaps antisocial activities is not deterred by the customs of his neighborhood peer group; it is all too easy for him to find a group with drives similar to his own. Furthermore, since the adolescent is intensely conscious of the mores of his selected peer group, his behavior tends to be an exquisite representation of the standards and expectations of the economic, social and cultural level of his associates.

The presenting problems of an adolescent patient may be the expression of a disorder in any of the diagnostic categories discussed in Chapter 8. The disturbance may be a continuation of a behavioral difficulty that developed in childhood, or it may appear for the first time in the adolescent period.

Unresolved Childhood Disturbances

Behavior problems that have not been resolved in childhood are likely to appear in intensified form in adolescence. For example, the boy who as a child was aggressively hostile may as an adolescent show overt hostility and direct it against a specific person. The girl who as a small child was so dependent she could not dress herself or go to school alone may carry along this dependency trait into adolescence and permit it to condition all her peer relationships. When childhood attributes of ingratiation, exploitation, arrogance, feelings of unworthiness, and other personality traits are carried over into adolescent life, their expression may have more serious and far-reaching effects.

The adolescent with a drive to ingratiate himself runs errands for his peers and older companions and does their bidding without regard for whether or not the commissions he executes are legitimate. The youngster who feels inadequate brags to cover up his lack of self-esteem or withdraws and is afraid to speak in class. The arrogant adolescent flaunts his knowledge and also his ignorance, and ridicules younger children when they make mistakes.

While normal adolescents may show an inclination to experiment with homosexual activity, evidences of a pathologic homosexuality may also emerge in adolescence and have overt manifestations. Sometimes homosexual activity or indications of identification with the opposite sex are clearly observed in adolescents who in childhood had apparently not revealed such tendencies, but earlier symptoms of homosexuality can usually be uncovered in a thorough exploration of the childhood history.

Learning difficulties which were perhaps considered unimportant in the informal setting of the lower school grades show up sharply in adolescence. They become a handicap in the more demanding atmosphere of high school with its impersonal departmental structure. The adolescent with unresolved learning difficulties may be overwhelmed by feelings of inadequacy and hopelessness, and may now take refuge in avoidance, clowning, defiance and other cover-up reactions.

While adolescence may exacerbate certain problems that existed earlier, these same difficulties may also disappear because as the youngster grows older he is able to find solutions that he could not arrive at before. Some conflicts at the root of preadolescent behavior and personality disturbances are resolved in adolescence, apparently because the necessary stimulus or motivation for change, previously lacking, is provided at this time. In the same way, some disturbances not amenable to treatment in childhood because no motivation could be aroused are responsive to therapy in adolescence.

The boy who as a preadolescent isolated himself and took no part in peer group activities as a protection against his feelings of social inadequacy may now be stimulated by his heterosexual drives to do something about his basic difficulties. The child who has dominated his family by tantrums may find that his adolescent companions are unmoved by these tactics. When the secondary gains of tantrums no longer exist, he may for the first time have a motivation for examining his customary way of behaving and be willing to attempt to change it. The adolescent girl who as a child had clung to dependency and its rewards may discover that to function independently brings greater satisfactions of a kind she had never before envisaged. Similarly, the obese child may in adolescence find stimulus for change in the urgent desire for social acceptance.

Disturbances Arising in Adolescence

A number of factors may give rise to problems peculiar to the adolescent period. These include the physical changes of puberty and the accompanying stresses, the fact that physiologic and psychologic development do not necessarily proceed at the same pace, and special environmental circumstances.

Pubertal Stress Situations

The age at which puberty begins and the pace at which the physical changes of puberty take place vary widely. In girls, menstruation and the beginning of breast development and axillary and pubic hair growth may appear as early as the ninth year or as late as the sixteenth. The girl with an early onset of puberty may find herself in close contact with older girls who are sophisticated while she is still a "little girl" emotionally. The girl with a markedly late onset of puberty may suffer from agonizing feelings of inferiority because she looks less mature than her peers; she must endure the disparaging comments on the lack of breast development so frequently made by both boys and girls. A youngster who has not yet begun to menstruate long after her companions have had this experience has vague apprehensions about her ability to marry and bear children, which she may be unwilling or unable to discuss with anyone.

In boys, the signs of puberty—the change of voice from treble to bass, the appearance of hair on the face and body, and the ability to have an erection—appear at various ages from eleven to sixteen. An early voice change is no handicap to a boy, but a late change is. The boy who still has a treble voice in his middle or late teens is likely to be taunted by his peers and called a homosexual in the various terms used by boys. Similarly, a boy who has to shave at an early age is rather envied, but delay in the appearance of hair is considered shameful. And in the many situations in which boys undress in company and compare their penises for size, the boy who is not mature enough to have an erection feels threatened and defenseless among peers who tend to regard an erection as the absolute measure of manhood. He is made to feel sexually inferior and may be unable to overcome this feeling in later life.

Physical and psychologic development do not always keep pace with one another; young boys and girls may be physically mature long before they are socially mature or sexually interested in the opposite sex. At varying ages and in varying degree, the adolescent becomes interested in establishing boy-girl relationships. For some adolescents this interest develops gradually and represents a continuation of the boy-girl relationships of early childhood with an ever-deepening emotional content. For others, the transition from childhood to adolescent boy-girl relationships is not so smoothly made. There are false starts, pretenses about not caring, rebuffs because of social awkwardness. The desire to be accepted by the peer group may drive adolescent boys and girls into sexual experimentation before their interest in heterosexual relationships warrants it or before they are emotionally mature enough for this experience.

The discrepancy that often exists between physical and psychologic development must also be kept in mind in judging the "fitness" of a youngster's behavior. If a youngster does have a significant deviation from the group in his physical maturation, one must be careful in deciding whether these features make the child seem more disturbed than he is (someone who "looks" the way he does shouldn't act the way he does) or actually do play a part in his underlying pathology.

External Stress Situations

Environmental circumstances that would not create stress in childhood may do so for the adolescent who is already vulnerable to the difficulties inherent in this period of life. The boy who was well adjusted as a child may as an adolescent be drawn into a group whose activities are antisocial; he may be "grown-up" enough to be a member of the group and yet not have the maturity needed for extricating himself from activities which he realizes are out of line with his basic values. The unsophisticated adolescent girl who formerly got on well socially may suddeny feel isolated if her peer group talks mainly about boys, dates and heterosexual relationships. Similarly, the sharply increased academic demands made upon the adolescent and the accelerated tempo of learning in high school may result in panic and self-questioning about innate ability in a youngster who has formerly managed quite well at school. Feelings of inadequacy and a lack of self-confidence may result in poor academic work and in dropping out of school.

Adolescents who differ from their peers in religion, race or social status may find themselves in stress situations that did not exist with these same companions in earlier years. As young people approach adulthood, they tend to conform more closely to the social patterns of their families than children do. This tendency affects their relationships with associates belonging to a minority group, whether racial or religious. The adolescent who belongs to a minority group may be shouldered out by his peers and isolated. He may be experiencing "prejudice" for the first time and be totally unprepared to handle it. Similarly, the youngster who comes from a mixed family in respect to race or religion may in adolescence gain his first sharp awareness of the social complications of his family background. Although such stressful situations are generally mastered with a resultant increase in maturity, this is not always the case.

An adoption situation may also be the focus of stress during this period of life. The adopted child who has not adequately comprehended the facts of adoption, or who is at odds with his adoptive parents, may be seriously disturbed in adolescence. All his vague doubts and confusions about his identity and security may boil up into intense conflicts, or he may become preoccupied with fantasies about his natural parents. Conversely, the nonadopted child may spin fantasies about being adopted in order to drive some harsh reality out of his consciousness.

Adolescence may also prove particularly stressful to children with special disabilities. These youngsters may suddenly find that their earlier adaptations do not work any more. Thus, the pressures of learning may prove too much for the mentally retarded child who made strides in learning to care for himself in earlier years; the new stimuli and demands of approaching maturity may overwhelm the youngster with cerebral dysfunction who heretofore successfully organized his environmental interactions. Similarly, the greater freedom of adolescence may make it impossible for a sociopathic youngster to keep his behavior in check any longer. The youngster with a physical handicap may now begin to feel like a social outsider.

Onset of Serious Disorders

Schizophrenia frequently appears for the first time in adolescence, although there may in individual cases be some question as to whether its onset at this time is a manifestation of previously unrecognized illness or a true beginning of the disorder. A significant proportion of epileptics have convulsions for the first time in adolescence. This disorder has serious psychologic repercussions. The first convulsions may have a shocking impact on the epileptic's peers, and his relationships with them are likely to be disrupted, particularly if convulsions continue for some length of time before they are controlled by medication. The adolescent epileptic may withdraw from social contacts, feeling that he cannot lead a normal life and that he will be unable to marry and have children.

Presenting Problems in Adolescence

The presenting problems in adolescence may give some clue to the severity of the disorder—but only a clue, since the child's over-all adjustment must be taken into account. There is no invariable correlation between the number and intensity of these problems and the seriousness of the underlying morbidity in terms of prognosis. Relatively minor complaints may be the precursors of incipient schizophrenia or of serious character disorders; numerous episodes of acting out may be only manifestations of transient situational stress. One youngster may experiment with drug-taking because he has gotten carried away with his peer group identification, but will stop as soon as he finds a better way to deal with the situation. Another youngster, however, takes drugs as part of his psychotic adjustment to life, and curing his addiction will be difficult or impossible. In the same manner, sexual experimentation by an adolescent cannot be categorized as a specific problem until it is understood in the context of his other behavior and the social mores.

Certain symptoms, however, occur with frequency among adolescents. These include suicide and anorexia nervosa, discussed earlier (see Chapter 11), and delinquency.

Delinquency

Far from being a clinical entity, the behavioral symptoms or disturbances commonly described as delinquent may figure in any of the personality patterns classified in Chapter 8, including those within the range of normality, despite the current popular tendency to ascribe common characteristics to all youngsters who commit unlawful acts. Delinquent behavior does not of itself brand a youngster as emotionally sick. Furthermore, individual psychiatric attention may not be his most pressing need if he is found to have some minor degree of psychopathology. For the child or adolescent whose antisocial acts represent an understandable reaction to acutely unfavorable environmental circumstances, psychiatric treatment may prove of little avail without a broader attack on basic social problems.

On the other hand, for the delinquent child who is emotionally disturbed, the fact of delinquency alone does not constitute a diagnosis or indicate the proper treatment. The type of therapy needed depends basically on the general diagnostic category to which the whole personality pattern belongs.

It is important to understand what is meant by delinquency. In the technical sense of the word it is the official entry in a court docket. Some of the outstanding works on the subject, among them the monumental studies of juvenile delinquents by Sheldon and Eleanor Glueck (1950), focus primarily on the legal aspects of the problem. Adherence to the primary definition makes it evident that it is not only how a person behaves but also the fact that some offensive act he commits leads to his apprehension and trial before an adjudicative tribunal that establishes his identity as a delinquent.

It is my belief that most delinquent acts are performed as part of a peer group activity in which the individual conscience of the youngster becomes dominated by his involvement with the group, the ideas of the group, or, in some cases, a kind of mass hysteria. Whether the act is called "juvenile delinquency" or "a youthful lark" often depends more on the youngster's socioeconomic class than on the objective nature of his behavior. Many college students go on a yearly rampage; often called a "panty raid," this is identified as delinquent behavior only rarely when there is a very large amount of property damage or if someone gets hurt. In contrast, the rampages of lower-class youngsters are usually considered delinquent gang fights, and only rarely viewed by the authorities as overspirited carrying-on that got out of hand. Thus, if two boys commit the same act of vandalism, one may become known as a delinquent by the usual process of judicial determination, whereas the other may escape being so branded because he acted on a college campus where his behavior was regarded as a prank. In still other cases, the distinction between delinquent and nondelinquent may arise from the family's ability to make good the damage done by the child.

Delinquency, therefore, is ultimately defined by a legal designation: the youngster has been apprehended and his act has been judged as delinquent and entered in the records as such. Any intervention that takes him off the hook as far as the actual recording is concerned makes him no longer delinquent. Thus, if the damage is undetected, if financial restitution is made, or if the judge releases the offender with a warning, the youngster can no longer legally be called delinquent, no matter what he has done.

However, for the present purposes, we will include among the "delinquents" those youngsters whose activities were not discovered and recorded.

While many delinquent youngsters have psychologic conflicts—often severe ones—these are not necessarily the reason for their antisocial behavior. Sometimes the connection between emotional difficulties and problem behavior is purely coincidental; in other words, they may be present simultaneously, like flat feet and a sore throat, but no cause-and-effect relationship can be established between them.

For some youngsters delinquent behavior is sociopathologic rather than psychopathologic in nature. For example, the delinquency may be the young person's way of adapting to his environment. He may live in a neighborhood where joining a gang is a matter of elementary precaution if he wants to come and go freely or seeks a gateway to acceptance by his peers. In some localities, both factors draw young people into activities that transgress the laws of the community. Nevertheless, adapting to a gang way of life is not the only social factor in delinquency. In a society where news reports of graft make clear that the community frequently closes its eyes to predatory activities and where adults often condone practices against which they preach, it is not to be wondered at that some young people acquire the idea that the real fault lies in being caught. Many striking parallels could be drawn between gang warfare among juvenile delinquents and the worldwide upheavals by which their elders settle their international disputes.

Children with behavior disorders may also participate in delinquent activities. For example, the child who suffers from a reactive behavior disorder is very likely to indulge somewhat experimentally in an occasional antisocial act, such as hurling a stone through a neighbor's window. He may make an adventure out of wandering through a department store and changing the price tag on any article he can lay his hands on. He may also do some petty shoplifting from time to time.

Although his characteristic actions have a strong nuisance value, the youngster with a reactive behavior disorder is not likely to come into sharp conflict with the law unless he happens to get caught up in the activities of an antisocial gang. Only on rare occasions or under unusually strong pressure from some more hardened associates does he take part in organized acts of violence or vandalism.

Delinquent children with neurotic behavior disorders, neurotic character disorders or psychoneuroses symbolically express their individual disturbances through their behavior. The antisocial acts of such a child will follow a pattern that indicates the nature of his problem. If his neurotic attitude is basically one of hostility, he may repeatedly hurl rocks through windows or engage in some other kind of apparently motiveless destruction. Sexual delinquency may be the mode of behavior through which he attempts to solve his conflicts. Stealing of objects which have the value of fetishes may be another form of symbolic expression. Neither jail sentences nor the imposition of fines on their parents will resolve the difficulties of youngsters whose conduct symbolically reflects such pathology. Their primary need is for psychiatric help. As their neurotic difficulties yield to the appropriate treatment, their behavior will tend to improve and hopefully they will be removed from the ranks of the delinquent. It should be noted that at present there are no data to indicate that neurotic youngsters form a higher proportion of the delinquent group than of the population at large.

In every assemblage of delinquents, one may find some psychotic children. A few are leaders and others are followers in the commission of antisocial acts. When a psychotic individual turns to crime, his activities may be bizarre and senselessly cruel, but, in other instances, it may be conspicuously ineffective. For example, a psychotic individual may stage a holdup at a store or a gas station, making it obvious that he does not have a dangerous weapon and allowing himself to be caught so easily that he quite clearly has not addressed himself to the issue of getting away free.

Though children in this group do not as a rule figure prominently in gang activities, glaring headlines every now and then report some brutal crime committed by one such child or a group led by a psychotic adolescent. When psychiatric examination of the brutal delinquent subsequently reveals that he had given prior indications of his pathologic condition, the public tends to respond with a hue and cry for the institutionalization of all grossly disturbed children as soon as their abnormal patterns of behavior are detected. Were such a policy to be put into effect, our already crowded correctional institutions would probably triple or quadruple their present populations; and many disturbed youngsters who are capable of overcoming their problems and leading lawful and productive lives in the open community would be deprived of the opportunity to do so. It is extremely difficult to determine if and when morbid preoccupations with hostility will erupt into antisocial acts; if every individual who showed such preoccupations were to be dealt with in the fashion suggested, a good proportion of our law-abiding population would now be behind locked doors. Nevertheless, more adequate psychiatric facilities for diagnosis and early treatment might prevent many disturbed youngsters from acting out their pathologic preoccupations.

Sociopathic youngsters represent a rather insignificant proportion of youthful offenders, even though they are often equated in the public mind with juvenile delinquents. The sociopath, who is typically impulsive and devoid of feelings of guilt or empathy, lacks the capacity to plan ahead or to function in a role of leadership for any significant period of time. Whether such a youngster becomes a harmless drifter or forms a pattern of delinquency is likely to be determined fortuitously by the social and economic circumstances of his life. Sociopaths who do become drawn into delinquent activities, usually under the influence of a stronger personality, are capable of committing flagrantly brutal and senseless acts in a conscienceless way.

Certain diseases of the brain impair judgment and render a child incapable of maintaining good control of his impulses. The youngster's irritability, hyperactivity and distractibility may interfere with his adjustment in school and stigmatize him in social situations. These characteristics also make him the prey of whatever peer group will accept him with all his defects. Denied recognition in other circles, he may get it by joining a gang of hoodlums. His presence there may be explained in part by the lack of adequate facilities for the constructive exploitation of his positive abilities. Individual acts such as stealing and fire-setting may also be perpetrated by youngsters whose high degree of impulsivity and lack of judgment are traceable to cerebral dysfunction.

The therapeutic handling that such a child requires is essentially the same as that indicated for nondelinquent children with similar dysfunction. In other words, treatment must focus on the basic organic problem. In some cases, the additional factor of sociologic distress has to be alleviated as far as possible. The hyperactive child living in cramped quarters may need additional living space before one can hope to guide his impulses into constructive channels.

Mentally retarded youngsters do not constitute an undue proportion of the delinquent group. Although the public tends to regard mentally defective youngsters as potential delinquents, those who come into conflict with the law represent a much smaller percentage of the total number of delinquents than the percentage of retardates in the total population.

Like the delinquent with an organic brain disease, the retardate who falls typically into some pattern of antisocial conduct becomes associated with a gang because other groups of his peers have failed to satisfy his need for social acceptance. Possessed of little judgment or ability to recognize the antisocial implications of his activities, he submissively performs any subordinate task delegated to him and obeys the commands of the more dominant personalities who exploit him. On his own, he may also engage in relatively minor forms of delinquency, such as purse-snatching.

The sexual delinquent in any diagnostic category may be a significant social problem if he habitually coerces younger or weaker children into engaging in heterosexual or homosexual acts.

A high correlation has been found to exist between learning difficulties and delinquency. Many young offenders fall into the category of poor readers. More than one child who begins to play hooky simply because of the misery arising from his poor scholastic performance, has fallen into the habit of spending the day with fellow truants who were devoting their time to some form of antisocial activity. Fearing to go home, the newcomer may join them in some petty theft in order to buy some food and he may gradually drift into other illegal activities.

Drug Abuse and Addiction

Drug addiction and intoxication spur many types of delinquent behavior. A distinction has to be made between the youth who uses drugs occasionally and the one who becomes addicted to them. The latter will go to extreme lengths of criminality to secure the wherewithal for drugs in order to prevent withdrawal symptoms. Since illegally sold drugs are often adulterated, there is the additional danger of toxic effects, particularly severe liver damage.

Alcohol is more commonly associated with rip-roaring gang activities. It has served to impair the judgment and stimulate the criminal activity of many gang recruits. They frequently share a bottle with their more hardened associates in order to demonstrate their manhood or to muster up the needed courage for some gang assignment for which they actually have little heart.

Diagnostic Considerations in Adolescence

The psychiatrist must attempt to estimate the psychodynamics underlying an adolescent's presenting problems without being unduly influenced by their superficial appearance and their impact on social values. In estimating the diagnostic implications of a compulsive trend, the important issue is not its effect on the milieu but its degree of inflexibility, its self-destructive character, and its possible indication of morbidity in the total behavioral pattern.

A fifteen year old boy who is unable to complete any assignment because his obsession with perfection prompts him to destroy school work whenever it falls short of that goal presents serious psychodynamic problems. So, too, does the boy who involves himself in frenetic sexual activity with older girls to prove his manhood, or runs away from home in an effort to start life on his own. The fact that treatment may take considerable time must be communicated to both family and patient.

Verbal Communication

The resolution of the adolescent's problems depends in some measure upon his capacity for verbal communication, upon whether it is difficult or easy for him to discuss his thoughts. Some adolescents appear to be eager to talk about their feelings and worries; if given the chance, they will explore their actions freely, accept interpretations, and show an amazing ability to be self-critical. Others hold back their words as if they were precious jewels to be bestowed only as a special favor. Such youngsters give the psychiatrist half-confidences; they cautiously test him, and then retreat into silence. They cannot unload their burden of worry even though they desperately want to do so. With these young patients a slight, almost meaningless revelation represents an enormous step forward in communication.

Still others do not verbalize their problems because they have no motivation for change. For example, a young boy's parents may be distressed at his late hours, but he sees no reason to answer for them, because to him his actions are merely a way of being left alone. A mother may complain that her daughter is rude and unobliging, keeps her room in a mess, and refuses to go along on family visits. The young girl—sometimes correctly—feels that she is holding her own in a battle of wills by taking the offensive. She has no motivation for giving up her habits or discussing them, since she considers them necessary tactics for self-preservation.

Discussion of Sexual Matters

In the treatment of adolescents, sexual matters are likely to be discussed since they are so important in this period of life. The psychiatrist should guard against interpreting all such issues as sexual preoccupation or conflict when they may merely be manifestations of peer rivalry expressed in terms of boy-girl relationships.

It should also be kept in mind that the terms used by adolescents to describe the sex organs and sexual acts change from generation to generation. The connotations of certain words also change and become more or less specific, milder or more forceful, and new words and phrases are used. The psychiatrist would do well to keep up to date in these matters. Inability to use the argot of a young patient in the sexual area may cut off free discussion. Conversely, the ability to do so may open up some hitherto closed area of confusion, doubt, or ambivalence for constructive scrutiny.

Diagnostic Approach

Although many adolescents are not interested in or even hostile to the idea of psychiatric consultation, very few refuse to participate in an initial interview. If the psychiatrist handles them with the courtesy and respect he would accord an adult, they will generally respond with courtesy and explain their attitudes and views. The teenager who feels that the psychiatrist wants to have his opinion of a specific problem will usually give it. He may protect himself by withholding information that would place him in a bad light, he may be suspicious and even hostile, but he usually gives his views.

The young patient's statements may be distorted by self-interest or by deep pathology, but this very act discloses useful material. The diagnostician's immediate objective is not to correct the patient's distortions but to get a clear understanding of his thought processes, distortions and point of view, and to gain insight about his ideas.

As indicated above, the adolescent patient should be handled more like an adult than a child. He should be made to feel that his unhappiness and conflicts are important because of their effect on him, not because of their effect on his parents. The presenting problem described by the parents may seem to have little relation to the problem as seen by the young patient. For example, the parents of an adolescent boy may report that he is rude and aggressively defiant of authority, and that his one asset is that he is sometimes acquiescent. The youngster will report that he is troubled by his inability to speak up when his rights are invaded—the very action considered an asset by the parents—and that when he is taken advantage of because of this inability he has a seething sense of outrage. He does not understand that his rudeness and defiance actually allow him to give vent to this sense of outrage, bursting forth at the wrong time and place and very likely against the wrong person.

In such situations the psychotherapeutic plan must be one of attack on the youngster's problem as he views it. Only after he has gained some understanding of the difficulty and begun to change can he face the issue of the impact of his behavior on others and their counter reactions.

As treatment gets under way, the adolescent should be approached as a responsible participant in his own case. The therapist should guard against becoming a partisan in a child-parent battle or creating the impression that he is one. The primary issue is always to work out the patient's psychiatric difficulties and his interpersonal problems. After these have been resolved, the patient will be able to communicate with his parents and, under ordinary circumstances, set up the kind of parent-child relationships which will facilitate the working out of most problems within the framework of the home.

In treating adolescents, the problem of acting out must be given special attention. The older the patient, the more his acting out may find expression in antisocial behavior, nuisance activities and self-destructive trends. The form which acting out takes may be a decisive factor in the tempo of treatment or in deciding that residential care with its safeguards is essential. If an adolescent reacts to anxiety with self-imposed starvation, accident proneness, running away from home, sexual promiscuity or suicidal attempts, his neurotic structure cannot be challenged adequately and safely outside of a residential treatment setting.

SELECTED REFERENCES

Aichhorn, A.: *Wayward Youth.* New York, Viking, 1935.

Ausubel, D. P.: *Theory and Problems of Adolescent Development.* New York, Grune & Stratton, 1954.

Chess, S.: Juvenile delinquency: whose problem? *Federal Probation,* Washington, June, 1955.

Connell, P. H.: Suicidal attempts in childhood and adolescence. *In* Howells, J. G. (Ed.): *Modern Perspectives in Child Psychiatry.* London, Oliver & Boyd, 1965.

Glueck, S., and Glueck, E. T.: *Unraveling Juvenile Delinquency.* New York, Commonwealth Fund, 1950.

Group for the Advancement of Psychiatry: *Normal Adolescence.* New York, Scribner's, 1968.

Jersild, A. T.: *The Psychology of Adolescence.* New York, Macmillan, 1963.

Tanner, J. M.: *Growth at Adolescence.* Springfield; Ill., Charles C Thomas, 1962.

Warren, W.: The psychiatry of adolescents. *In* Howells, J. G. (Ed.): *Modern Perspectives in Child Psychiatry.* London, Oliver & Boyd, 1965.

16. Psychotherapy and Related Treatments

MEDICAL SCIENCE has not blessed the child suffering from a behavior disorder with remedies that are as specific and fast-working as those available for controlling many physical ailments. The treatment of emotional difficulties is a much more highly individualized procedure. It must be planned with due regard for the complex interaction of factors in the origin and development of a child's problem. In many cases, pathologic aspects of the child's interpersonal relationships and life setting are of as much concern to the therapist as the immediate imprint of the disorder on the patient's personality.

Psychotherapy, which attempts to deal with these issues, must therefore be viewed in broad terms. Although many definitions have been offered, for purposes of the present discussion, psychotherapy will be considered to include any method of treatment that directly effects changes in a child's feeling and behavior patterns. It encompasses not only direct treatment of the child but also environmental manipulation and work with parents to effect constructive changes in a child's day-to-day living experiences. The child may be treated in a group or individually, in the setting of a private office or a large institution. Psychotherapy may be used exclusively or in conjunction with drugs. In general, it involves the communication of ideas and the satisfaction of emotional needs through specially structured interpersonal relationships or living experiences. Play and other activity appropriate to the youngster's age, sex and personal interests figure prominently in various forms of psychotherapy used with children.

Regardless of the form selected, certain general principles govern the administration of psychotherapy. How it is to be employed depends upon the nature of the basic pattern underlying the child's symptoms. Is this pattern reactive, neurotic, schizophrenic, sociopathic, or does it, rather, constitute impulsive hyperactivity due to cerebral dysfunction? After making the diagnosis, the therapist formulates a plan of treatment designed to alter or redirect the underlying pattern. The program should take into account the specific degree of alteration that would be desirable. In planning to modify a neurotic pattern, for example, it is important to distinguish between behavior that represents an overlay of neurosis and behavior that actually reflects the child's basic personality. Our aim is to change the caricature of personality, not its essence.

Parent Guidance

When a child is suffering from a reactive behavior disorder, a neurotic behavior disorder, or from some problem related to an environmental situation, parent guidance may be employed as either the primary or supplementary approach to his treatment. Counseling may also be indicated for parents of children with fixed pathology, such as mental retardation, organic behavior disorder, or some physical disability. A restructuring of parental demands will usually contribute to the alleviation of behavioral symptoms that may have developed secondary to the disorder.

The primary goal of a guidance program is to organize the parent's behavior in such a way as to provide the most constructive environment for the healthy development of the child. This implies a twofold aim: to eliminate those patterns of child-parent interaction that are exerting a deleterious influence, and to mobilize and expand those patterns that would have a healthy impact.

The decision to employ guidance in a given case assumes that the parents are capable of understanding and following the therapist's advice and that they are genuinely motivated to do so. The focus is on changing specific features of the parents' handling of the child or on modifying certain of their overtly expressed attitudes toward the child. No direct attempt is made to define or change any hypothetic underlying conflicts, anxieties or defenses in the parent which might (according to some theories of child behavior) be presumed to be the basis for their overtly expressed attitudes and thus the cause of the noxious behavior in the child. The presumption that *all* poor handling is the result of emotional disturbance in the parents, and that changes can be effected only through direct treatment of the parents' problems, is definitely

without basis in my experience. Again and again, very significant
changes in parental attitude and functioning toward the child
have occurred when the parent achieves a better understanding of
the child and his interaction with the environment.

Poor handling, in most cases, springs from less esoteric sources
than the parents' own emotional problems. Frequently parents
develop negative attitudes toward the child, not because of basic
rejection, but rather because of the child's overt problem behavior
and their inability to cope with it. They are confused about what
is causing the problem; their frustration at their own incompetence
and lack of power to control the child gives rise to displays of
anger and hostility, thus increasing the negative interaction and
in turn aggravating the symptoms; finally, feelings of guilt, reinforced by many prevalent theories on the origin of behavior disorders, lead to inconsistency.

This is not to imply that all parents are capable of responding
well to a counseling approach. There *are* parents who are seriously
disturbed, who overwhelmingly reject or are markedly ambivalent
toward the child; with these parents, obviously, guidance can be
of little avail. Moreover, recommendations may be carried out in
a manner so contradictory to their purpose that the problem may
be increased. In these situations it is necessary to seek an alternative
method of treatment. The child may have to be removed from the
home situation, if therapy alone is not sufficient, and the parent
should be advised to seek psychiatric help for himself.

The first step in guidance is to give the parents an understanding
of the dynamics of the child's problem and why special handling
is required. The therapist should identify those factors in the
child's behavior that are due to his basic temperament, or to organic
causes. Within this frame of reference, the parents should be
helped to recognize which demands have been inappropriate and
have been having a harmful effect. These demands may have been
unrealistic because the parents were unaware of the norms for
children in general and had overly high expectations. On the other
hand, the demands may not have been excessive in themselves but
in relation to a particular child's temperamental characteristics
or his physical or intellectual limitations. The parents should be
shown in what way these demands have created stress for the child,
and should be given concrete suggestions as to how these demands

must be modified in order to improve their relationship with the child.

Giving the parents general prescriptions to change their behavior is insufficient. Rather, they must be shown in detail and with examples how their handling of the child can be made appropriate. Concrete incidents in the child's life which clarify and illustrate various points in the program should be interwoven into all discussions to make sure the parents understand the advice.

Guidance of this sort may be given on a single occasion and have a therapeutic effect on the child. But it may be necessary to plan periodic discussions with the parents, especially if they find it difficult to give up their expectations of the child. Since the specific expression of the child's limitations may vary as he grows older, it is often useful to plan sessions with the parents to explain these fluctuations. In some cases, it is best to have a series of closely spaced discussions so as to cover rather quickly the areas about which the parents are puzzled or are behaving inappropriately. With this format, new ways of handling the child are suggested for each incident mentioned by the parents, who then report back to the adviser what they attempted and how it worked or didn't work. In this way the psychiatrist can see almost immediately whether the parents have comprehended his recommendations.

In general, it is advisable to include both parents in the guidance sessions whenever possible, especially at the beginning. No program can be successful unless it is understood by the major parties who are to carry it out. If either parent has doubts, questions or misunderstandings, he can best clear these up by being an active participant in the guidance program. Of course, if an interim discussion will involve the minutiae of the mother's handling of certain aspects of the child's daily life, only she need be present. However, this should not be made into the permanent plan. There are some instances in which group guidance may be more effective than individual discussions. When several parents have the same type of problem with their children, they experience some relief at hearing that other parents have similar difficulties. At other times, the way one parent handles a problem may give another parent an idea about his own actions, whether this be a positive or negative influence. Some parents who are shy when alone with the psychiatrist may be emboldened when they hear other mothers or fathers discussing their problems and their child-care methods. Obviously, to have a successful group arrangement one must organize the members carefully; the discussions will not be therapeutic if one parent monopolizes the session or attacks the others.

As a rule, behavior imposed on a parent who has no attitudinal basis for it will be maintained only as long as direct pressure is being exerted on him. Nevertheless, sufficient respect for the authority—not authoritarianism—of the professional guiding the situation, or sufficient despair over a situation so that a parent is willing to try something new, may motivate him to accept demands imposed upon him. And, in many instances, concern about the development of the child can cause a parent to make substantial alterations in his handling even if his basic attitudes remain contrary to the child's best interests. Frequently, the improvements in the child's behavior that follow may move the parent to reassess his attitudes.

Any failure by the parent to comply with recommendations made should be regarded as a problem to be analyzed rather than as justification for a reproachful reaction on the part of the counselor. The psychiatrist should never act as if he blames the parents for the child's disorder. Rather, his approach is to treat the parents as allies, even as colleagues, in the therapy of the child. The parents want suggestions and information and need to be redirected, not castigated. Even if they have little or no real emotional understanding of their child's problems, parents who experience some personal gain from the suggestions made early in the counseling process may then prove willing to cooperate in the child's treatment on a long-range basis.

Parent guidance is an effective therapeutic technique with children in most of the diagnostic categories. Its use with youngsters who have reactive behavior disorders is obvious: the aim is to correct the situation which is proving stressful to the child. Children with neurotic behavior disorders may also be treated in this way, especially in those situations where direct psychotherapy will not work either because the child does not evidence his problem in a therapeutic situation, or because he doesn't recognize that he has any problem and therefore cannot even talk about it. Similarly, appropriate programming through parent guidance may be a way of obtaining the optimum adaptation from a child with schizophrenia or cerebral dysfunction.

In the New York Longitudinal Study, parent guidance was used as the initial therapeutic procedure with children who developed a behavior problem. In almost half of the cases the parents showed marked or moderate changes in behavior in the direction suggested by the psychiatrist, and there was recovery or marked or moderate improvement in the children. This success has been duplicated in my private and clinic patients with a variety of psychiatric problems and from diverse sociocultural backgrounds. As a therapeutic method, parent guidance has also proved to be highly efficient. Significant improvement in a child's behavior was reported after an average of only 2.3 guidance sessions in the longitudinal study. In private and clinical practice, the number of sessions required has been about two to four times greater, but this is still markedly less than would have been required for any other psychotherapeutic procedure.

Play Therapy

The purely verbal form of communication employed in the psychotherapeutic treatment of an adult is, of course, of limited value in the treatment of a child. While discussion may represent a desirable therapeutic approach to adolescents, as well as some preadolescents and younger children, play or handicraft activity affords a more natural means of communication for most children. Through such activity, a child displays his typical behavior, attitudes to people, and manner of tackling issues. His defensive behavior patterns are also delineated, albeit to a rather restricted degree.

Although it is now used by therapists with diverse theoretic approaches, play therapy has often been regarded as synonymous with child psychoanalysis because it was first dispensed as a systematic technique within that framework. Over the years, however, play therapy has gradually been elevated to its present status as a specific therapeutic technique at the disposal of any psychotherapist, regardless of his orientation. It is generally recognized today as an invaluable method of dealing with young children.

Whether employed in child analysis or in nonanalytically oriented treatment, play represents a favorable medium for the spontaneous expression of feelings, thoughts, and conflicts—in a disguised fashion, if necessary. Play also permits, indeed encourages, free motility. This is important in the therapeutic session, since most children become extremely uncomfortable if they are kept still for long periods of time.

During play therapy, the psychiatrist may choose to be primarily supportive or to stress interpretation. He may devote himself to building up a good relationship, or he may structure the interviews for encouraging emotional release. The attitudes which he expresses through what he does and how he does it may be at least as important as the ideas he puts into words.

In private practice, play therapy is usually administered to a patient from one to three times weekly. In the child guidance clinic, play sessions are generally scheduled once a week.

The effective use of play as a therapeutic device requires thoughtful planning of setting and facilities. The playroom itself should be a pleasant one, furnished simply and practically. Any object that might easily be damaged or soiled would be out of place in the room, which ideally should contain a low sink and a floor covered in tile, linoleum or some other easily washable material. Smocks should be available for the children and therapist to slip into, whenever their activity involves water, paints or clay.

Toys and play materials appropriate for children of all ages and tastes should be provided. Elaborate or complicated articles, such as mechanical playthings whose operation would completely absorb a youngster's attention, do not belong in the therapy playroom. With these exceptions, the assortment may include anything that would be within the child's capacity to use creatively, would hold his attention long enough to demonstrate what can be accomplished through application, and would contribute to the formation of a good relationship, or facilitate the structuring of a situation in a particular way.

For the very young child, blocks, fire engines and other toy autos and trucks should be available, as well as dolls and a doll house with toy furniture and some play food.

Assorted toy guns, dart guns, balls, balloons, toy soldiers and a punching bag are other standard items. A few competitive games such as checkers, Chinese checkers and dominoes may be useful. Books are brought into the playroom when they seem suitable.

Graphic media should be well represented. Pencils, crayons, paints and clay ought to be available, along with an ample supply of plain and colored paper. It is well to provide a blackboard with plenty of chalk. Craft materials, such as those for making leather objects, model airplanes or jewelry, can also be put to good use.

A suitable activity usually suggests itself in the course of the diagnostic work-up, especially in the initial session. Taking advantage of the clues provided, one may permit the child, during the early phase of therapy, to determine his own activity and the length of time he will continue it. He thus provides us with a definition of his spontaneous level of activity. It is on this definition that the planned approach to the alteration of his behavior should be based.

The mere continuation of the activity cannot be regarded as therapy, for only in a relatively few cases does this lead to a constructive change in behavior, attitudes and emotions. More than the presence of an adult called "therapist" is necessary to bring about desirable changes. At this stage, the child's activity should be structured in accordance with a definite plan.

The therapist must organize the play with two major purposes in mind: to gain understanding of the child's problems as these are expressed symbolically or directly through his playroom activities, and to bring about desirable changes in the child's behavior.

The initial interview sets the stage and is of crucial importance for the entire treatment process. Even if the child is on his best behavior, his conduct and attitudes during this session frequently constitute a surprisingly accurate portrayal of his major psychologic defenses, as often becomes evident when the session is later reviewed. An undercurrent of suspiciousness, or such attitudes as overcompliance, carelessness or uncritical friendliness, may become apparent from a study of the first session.

Brief interchanges from an initial interview will illustrate the point. Charles, an eight year old boy, entered the playroom with a backward glance at his mother. Invited to look over the play materials and decide which he'd like to use, Charles stood stiffly as he remarked, "I'll make a picture." (Do you want to use paints or crayons?) "I don't think my mother wants me to paint. I might get my shirt dirty." (Suppose we ask her.) When we returned to the waiting room and put the question to Mrs. B., she answered,

"Certainly you may paint. We can wash out the paint if it gets on your clothes." Back in the playroom, Charles glanced irresolutely at the paint jars and then at the box of crayons. "What do you think I should use?" (They're both fun. Whichever you decide.) "I think I'll crayon."

The boy's incorporation into his own personality of a compulsive cleanliness characteristic of his mother, despite her willingness in that situation to modify her attitude, became evident at the very opening of the initial interview. This turned out to be one of the central problems that had to be resolved in treatment. Similarly, the boy's great need to rely on the authority of an adult and his ultimate selection of a medium that could be rigidly controlled, which also became an important issue in the case, were manifested in this early treatment situation.

As psychotherapy proceeds, each interview or group of interviews should build on what was accomplished during the preceding sessions, so that details of the child's symptoms, his mode of forming interpersonal relationships, and his system of behavioral defenses are constantly being unfolded. The nature of the activity may vary from one session to the next, or the same type of play or project may continue for a number of sessions.

Patterns of motor activity generally tend to dominate the early sessions and then to be overshadowed by the symbolic content of the play as the therapy facilitates the communication of thoughts, attitudes and feelings. During this process, the therapist's participation in the play, the degree of activity or passivity he manifests, and his specific approach to his young patient will be determined by his own theoretic orientation and goals, by the nature of the problems to be resolved, and by what is required to form a good emotional relationship with a particular child.

Irrespective of these factors, certain pointers may prove helpful. A completely permissive attitude is of limited application in the playroom. To effect constructive change, it is almost always necessary to exert some pressure on a child for behavior different from what would occur spontaneously. For example, one may press for just a bit more concentration and sustained effort than is characteristic of a youngster's functioning. At times, too, it may become important to aid and encourage him by making his handiwork appear to be more successful than usual. This may be done by making unreported repairs or improvements between sessions in some object he has been creating. The clearing away of all materials or toys except those with which it is desired that the child busy himself during a session may serve to facilitate the release of hidden feelings.

A situation may be structured either to limit activity or to impose demands for a kind of activity different from what a child would engage in of his own accord. One may wish an overclean, compulsive youngster to experience unstructured or messy play. A request for better workmanship from a child who usually turns out hastily nd poorly executed plane models may lead to new types of experience for him and to the development of more favorable attitudes. When the tempo of progress appears to be slowing down, some planned activity may give the incentive needed for further change.

Activity during play therapy often gives rise to meaningful discussions, provided that due allowance is made for the limits which a child's age imposes on his ability to conceptualize. One of the best subjects for these discussions is the child's dreams.

Utilization of Dreams

The study and interpretation of dreams can shed much light on a child's thoughts and feelings, and he should be encouraged to report them. Dreams may provide significant clues to the nature of obscure conflicts and fears, or to the identity of those with whom the dreamer's relationships are disturbed. Wishes that he is unable to reveal or satisfy during his waking hours are often directly fulfilled by his mind during sleep. Other dreams constitute disguised representations of ambivalent impulses and problems that he expresses but fails to resolve through his symptoms.

Anxiety dreams are not uncommon in youngsters. Their manifest content generally betrays the level of cognition achieved by the dreamer, as well as the environmental forces impinging upon him. More than one fearful child has dreamt of burglars at his bedroom door or of being devoured by lions. His sleep may also be troubled by visions of black widow spiders, of being trapped or plunging downward in an elevator, or of cowering before a witch who has driven his mother from home.

Such dreams can be as productive of meaningful associations as those of the adult. Their examination during therapy sessions may strikingly illuminate almost forgotten traumatic incidents, consciously denied negative feelings toward a parent, or fallacious connections drawn between temporally coincidental events. The analysis and timely interpretation of such material, in whatever terms will be most meaningful for the child, will facilitate his understanding of his difficulties.

Dreams pointing to the resolution of conflicts are indicative of therapeutic progress and emotional growth, especially if they come to represent a child's predominant dream state. Reappearing in them in a less terrifying way may be images and scenes that figured in the anxiety dreams. The lions, for example, may now be envisioned as friendly denizens of the local zoo, while any burglar bold enough to return will perhaps be routed by a night watchman or alert stranger. The stranger may eventually be recognized as the dreamer's father; he may also shoo away the ugly witch so that mother may assume her rightful place at the breakfast table.

Daydreams, products of a different state of consciousness and functioning, do not duplicate those which come with sleep. Nevertheless, they merit exploration and discussion, for they, too, yield significant clues to a youngster's hopes, fears and problems. Since children tend to feel more responsible for their fantasies than for their mental productions during sleep, disclosures of the former are more likely to be censored, particularly if the therapist is expected to disapprove of them. It is well to bear in mind that fantasies are generally reported less fully and reliably than dreams.

When the child brings into the treatment situation behavioral and verbal communication expository of his relationship with the main figures in his life, this is technically known as transference. Its development enables the therapist to examine and define with greater exactitude a youngster's unhealthy attitudes and defenses as well as his positive personality attributes. The necessary modifications can then be facilitated by providing him with the new types of interpersonal experience that he needs, and by helping him through timely and appropriate interpretation. Eventually, the time comes for the therapist to begin to criticize the child's psychologic defenses or discuss the dynamics involved. He always does so, of course, in terms corresponding to the patient's own conceptualizations, which vary from age to age. When the youngster later begins to criticize his own behavior, his treatment may be said to be in its final phase.

Release Therapy

A highly specific and primarily cathartic form of play therapy—termed "release therapy"—has been suggested by David Levy (1939). He points out that the normal small child resorts to imaginative play to rid himself of tensions created by his emotional difficulties. If, for some reason, he is unable to do this, the symptoms which indicate the presence of his disturbance tend to become manifest.

Throwing, cutting, hitting, spilling water on the floor, and similar activities that present opportunities to release aggression and reexperience infantile pleasures characterize this type of treatment. The therapist makes minimal use of interpretation, since it is assumed that the release afforded by the child's activity will resolve his tensions.

This form of therapy is suitable for normal children with certain recurrent problems, as well as for disturbed youngsters. Release therapy may be useful for a child who needs to express his fears after undergoing a frightening experience, such as witnessing a serious accident. It also helps a timid child who is constantly being bullied.

Whatever the type of activity, according to Levy, the therapist should assume these two important responsibilities: to prevent the acting-out behavior from endangering either the child or himself; and to make certain that the youngster does not leave the session under the impression that the therapist is encouraging similar acting-out behavior at home or elsewhere.

Art Therapy

Art plays a therapeutic as well as a diagnostic role in child psychiatry. This medium is especially valuable with youngsters who find it hard to express their thoughts and feelings in words or in play. Art may also serve to facilitate the disclosure of an emotionally charged idea by a child who generally has no difficulty in using other forms of communication. If he is too apprehensive to talk about a frightening dream, for example, he may be able to express its content in a drawing.

The youngster should be provided with a generous assortment of drawing materials so that he may select those with which he can express himself most freely. His choice of medium is itself very revealing. The spontaneous child usually prefers materials that cannot be rigidly controlled, such as fingerpaints. The compulsive child is likely to feel most at home with crayons or pencils. The former, however, may use crayons in a delightfully imaginative way, while the compulsive child would tend to use fingerpaints mechanically.

In order to determine dominant trends, a number of productions should be examined. A comparative study of the maturity of approach, the choice of subject matter, and the materials used in a series of pictures drawn during the course of therapy provides a graphic record of a child's progress.

Relationship Therapy

The foremost advocate of relationship therapy in the American child guidance movement was Frederick H. Allen (1942), who described this treatment approach in *Psychotherapy with Children*.

Instead of emphasizing unconscious drives and instinctual gratification, Allen's interpretations focus on what a child's behavior in a session demonstrates about his relationship with his therapist. The child's initial responses must be used regardless of their content, he emphasizes, "to establish a relationship that will help the child develop to a more creative and responsible acceptance of himself." Because he believes that such a relationship has a much greater therapeutic value than an understanding of the past which molded the child's present behavior, Allen relegates historical data to a position of minor importance.

The search for content in discussions with a child, according to Allen, may side-track the therapeutic process from the more important goal of helping the youthful patient gain the freedom to talk and therefore to share his thoughts and feelings with another person. As Allen points out, "The therapist who is preoccupied with eliciting a particular content, who leaps with eager zeal to each word connected with that content, frequently puts a force into the relationship that makes it more difficult for the child to get to the point of actual sharing." While few psychiatrists today would use relationship therapy as an exclusive modality, it plays a very important part in all types of treatment.

Group Therapy

The psychotherapeutic techniques described above, though developed for the treatment of individuals, may also be administered to groups of children, adolescents or parents. In addition, special techniques have been developed specifically for group work, such as the concept of activity group therapy originally described by S. R. Slavson (1950).

Whether it uses general or special psychotherapeutic techniques, group therapy is not merely a way of increasing a psychiatrist's patient load by permitting him to see several children in the time normally allotted to one. Rather, this approach should be used when it is specifically appropriate for a given child. Group therapy may sometimes be used diagnostically. For example, a child may have difficulties in his peer relationships which may not show up as clearly in the patient-therapist situation as they do in the group. Similarly, a highly distractible child may respond to the structured stimuli of an individual therapy session in an organized and orderly fashion, whereas when he is confronted with the distracting influences of other children and the many sounds, sights and activities of a group, he displays his more characteristic disorganized and highly active behavior. If the therapist were only to see him alone, he would learn very little about the youngster's problem and its underlying dynamics. However, if he introduces the child into an organized group whose functioning is structured but nevertheless presents many different stimuli to the child, he may be able to discern the origins of the difficulty.

For some children a group situation may be best for treatment as well as for diagnosis. For example, placing the distractible child described above in the situation where one already knows that he functions well does nothing to increase his ability to function in troublesome situations. Only in a group will the problems present themselves in a way that enables the therapist to interpret them to the child, refocus his behavior, or gather knowledge on which to base his suggestions for appropriate environmental changes. Similarly, the group context is most helpful in handling the child who is aggressive with his peers but not with adults, or the child who is obsequious and characteristically defers to his peers.

Before placing a child into a group, however, the therapist must understand the nature of his individual problem and work out a therapeutic plan for him. It is usually necessary, therefore, to have separate sessions with each child beforehand so as to establish a relationship with him. Then, when the child has entered the group, the therapist is prepared to intervene, interpret actions, and suggest solutions that not merely restore peace or maintain a sense of fair play in the group as a whole, but also enhance each child's own direction of growth and decrease his neurotic or maladaptive patterns. Even during the course of group therapy, it may be best for the psychiatrist to meet with a child independently when he feels that individual discussion would be therapeutic.

The therapist must choose the participants in a group with care. Whether the group is to consist of preschool or school-age children, preadolescents or adolescents, there should be a balance of personalities. To gather a group composed only of disorganized children would be to have the experience of their disorganization multiplied by the number of youngsters, thus enhancing the disorder of each child by the effect of the others. This would obviously not be a therapeutic group. Similarly, an assemblage of several well-behaved, inhibited children might not be a bad therapeutic unit, but it would take a great deal more effort and time on the part of the leader than if the group included some more assertive children as a kind of balance.

In general, it is best to have a diversity of diagnostic categories represented in a group. If this is not practicable, then it is a good idea to include children with different symptoms, even if, let us say, they are all diagnosed as having neurotic behavior disorders. Naturally, there will be exceptions to this rule. It may, for example, be best to group together children who are suffering from the same organic disease or who have similar worries. Ironically, these often turn out to be rather heterogeneous groups since each youngster's troubles may represent a different adaptation—normal, reactive or neurotic.

A group should consist of at least four children—with three there is usually the danger that one will become the scapegoat of the others. How the group will be organized usually depends upon the age of the children. Preschool children are generally organized as an activity group. The therapist gives the youngsters play materials through which they can develop appropriate attitudes and relationships. In this age group, interpretation plays a minor role. Group therapy can enhance the young child's independence and alleviate separation anxiety through fostering gradual transfer of his faith in his mother to the therapist.

With somewhat older children, activity would probably be the major therapeutic modality, but more discussion can be expected to take place. Depending upon the competence of the group, one might include craftwork or even trips.

In a group of preadolescents or adolescents, discussion may become the predominant modality, but the therapist may still use various activities to channel the children's energies, so that they are not called upon just to sit and talk. How an activity is set up will depend upon the therapist's talents and the children's desires. For example, the girls in a group with which I was once involved wanted to sew. I was able to bring in material and worked along with them. During the sessions they began to feel they were creating something worthwhile; at the same time, the project was a way of achieving independence. They found they could take criticism of what they were doing, first in sewing and then in other areas, and that this could be a constructive as well as a destructive experience. They also became aware that they sometimes asked for help merely as a way of controlling the therapist's attention, and they learned to distinguish between such requests and those based on a genuine need for assistance. Later they were able to generalize these findings from their sewing experience and apply them in their day-to-day living.

The specific activity may vary considerably so long as it is being used therapeutically. Certain activities do not lend themselves to this purpose. Thus, chess is not a practical game for an activity group: a youngster calculating his moves is unlikely to discuss his inner thoughts. One must avoid having a child become so involved with the intricate rules of a game that he is easily able to set up a barricade against interpersonal relationships.

Group therapy is a demanding technique. One must be on guard against permitting the activity to become merely that of a recreation group. Slavson tends to assume that if the children are properly chosen, their individual ways of behaving will modify each other in a therapeutic way with little intervention by the psychiatrist. I believe that the therapist must become more involved. He must give direction to the group in order to insure that its activity is an effective vehicle for therapy. He must keep the group cohesive, while mobilizing the positive qualities of each individual.

Sometimes, adolescents or preadolescents will do better with group therapy oriented to discussion rather than activity. Qualifying for membership in a discussion group would be youngsters who were consciously dissatisfied with their own conduct, or, at least, with their interpersonal relationships, and who had the intellectual capacity to explore verbally their own behavior and motivations and those of the other youngsters. The therapist leading such a group would make clear that its participants were coming together to investigate and solve their personality problems. A self-critical attitude would not be demanded of youngsters entering the group, although hopefully it should emerge. A meaningful airing of problems and general participation are facilitated when the group members are about the same age.

Family Therapy

In the past decade, family therapy has become established as a separate form of psychiatric treatment. This approach is based on the concept that the child's attitudes and behavior are largely derived from or demonstrated in familial interaction. The therapeutic effort is directed toward identifying and changing the unhealthy relationships of the patient to the rest of the family as well as such relationships of other members of the family toward one another.

Typically, the entire family unit is gathered for each session. Anything that is said and done during the session may become a topic for discussion. In addition, the therapist may bring up other subjects he deems pertinent. There is in fact wide variation in the choice of topics and the manner in which they are commented upon. Children may be strongly encouraged to make critical comments about their parents and complaints about sibs. Discussion about sexuality may include inquiry into the sexual practices of the parents, with interpretations of hidden hostilities or derogations. In the most extreme form of this free family interchange, the therapist's attitude may be a strong signal to the child patient and his sibs that parental authority is superseded and to be met with contempt. Whether this is of therapeutic value may indeed be questioned in many cases.

If sensitively used, however, family therapy may make it possible for both child and parents to become clear about previously obscure attitudes and habits of thought. With this insight, a speedier redressing of grievances is sometimes possible. Parents who are capable of being allies of the therapist may also be given a quicker and clearer exposition of those changes in their behavior and attitudes that will be beneficial to the child.

Many family therapists utilize a flexible approach, identifying certain topics as suitable for exploration privately with one or both parents without the children, or with the child patient free from the exposure of a sensitive point to the gibes of his brothers and sisters. Thus, there may be sessions with any combination of family members for as many times as appear useful in pursuing the therapeutic goal.

There can be no question that the proper practice of child psychiatry should include interviewing all family members necessary for defining the dynamics of the behavioral pathology. Therapy, too, should include those family members whose attitudes and activities are perpetuating the youngster's noxious self image and behavioral traits. It is therefore appropriate to consider one or a series of group discussions which include the child and one or more family members, or various combinations of family members without the child. A number of psychiatrists have utilized these procedures for many years, even though it is only recently that they have been labeled as family diagnosis and therapy. Other psychiatrists have clung to the concept that the therapist can be the patient's advocate only if he remains rigorously out of contact with other members of the family. This traditional view has always been of dubious merit. Only those who accepted it in the past now find it necessary to invoke a new therapeutic title, "family therapy," to justify the abandonment of this view.

Behavior Therapy

Based essentially on learning theory, behavior therapy uses the techniques of conditioning. These include classic conditioning, operant conditioning, counterconditioning and extinction.

As defined by Eysenck (1959) and Wolpe (1958), behavior therapy categorizes behavior disorders as "maladaptive behaviors" rather than "psychopathology." The presenting symptoms do not reflect an underlying disorder; the symptoms themselves constitute the illness. Therefore, elimination of the symptoms is cure.

While the theory is vigorously disputed by many, the techniques of behavior therapy are widely used by psychiatrists and psychologists. Many clinicians find that certain symptoms are so troublesome that, even if they are assumed to represent an underlying conflict, their eradication is desirable as a first step toward more normal functioning. Increasingly, residential centers are using behavior therapy techniques in treating severely retarded and schizophrenic children.

In clinical practice, behavior therapy has been used most successfully to eliminate phobias, such as animal or school phobia, and to overcome age-inappropriate behaviors, such as enuresis or tantrums. The therapist treats phobias by means of deconditioning. After setting up a hierarchy of stimuli graded according to the strength of the phobic reaction, the clinician works out a series of deconditioning situations. Initially, the patient is exposed to circumstances that evoke milder aspects of his phobic reaction, coupled with a pleasurable event. With repetition of this experience and decreasing phobic reaction, the patient is exposed to increasingly severe stimuli in the same manner until the phobic symptom has been eliminated.

In other cases, the therapist creates a desired conditioned reflex to correct such specific behaviors as enuresis. One illustration of this technique is the use of electrical devices for wakening the child when he starts to wet the bed. With repetition of this sequence the child finally becomes conditioned to awaken in response to the sensation of a full bladder. He is rewarded by the awareness that he no longer has to be embarrassed by bedwetting.

In a broad review, Werry and Wollersheim (1967) conclude that "behavior therapy with children, though no panacea, seems likely to bring limited but significant relief at least to certain patients presently unamenable to, or unreachable by, traditional techniques."

Choosing Therapeutic Methods and Goals

Diagnosis is usually the principal guide to treatment. It provides the direct evidence about the etiology and nature of the child's disorder and points to the treatment of choice for its cure or alleviation. But in many cases practical considerations have to be taken into account. If the treatment of choice requires therapeutic skills and facilities that are not available in the community, the actual selection is dictated in large measure by what the community does have to offer. The cost of treatment is another determining factor. Since intensive individual psychotherapy is generally lengthy and expensive, the economic resources of the youngster's family may make it necessary to recommend another method.

In setting his goals for the treatment of the child, the therapist may choose from a broad spectrum of possibilities. These range from constructive channeling of disturbed thinking to complete reversal of the underlying emotions and attitudes. The choice of goals and method of therapy will depend in large measure on the therapist's estimate of the degree of pathology present and the reversibility of the defense patterns, the patient's age, intellectual level and motivation to change, as well as on his family's ability to examine and alter their own attitudes and other detrimental environmental influences.

Since goals play a vital part in the over-all planning of a case, they must be set early in treatment. But a flexible approach is required; goals have to be revised as evidence begins to accumulate that the degree of pathology is less or greater than had been anticipated. Children are often on their best behavior in their early sessions with the therapist; hence, some time may elapse before the behavior suggested as typical in the presenting problems can be confirmed and evaluated through clinical observation. In addition to the over-all goals, the therapist also sets a succession of intermediate goals. These reflect the therapeutic factors being stressed at each phase of treatment, based on the progress already made.

Terminating Treatment

Criteria for terminating treatment vary. Some mirror the limited goals that had to be set for a particular case. The reports that a child is functioning well in all situations, and notably in the problem areas, suggest that his treatment may be nearing termination If the therapist's observations tally with these reports, treatment should be brought to a close. In other instances, the signal for ending treatment is that the child has reached a plateau on which he is functioning about as well as he can be expected to perform in view of the diagnostic picture. Termination of a case is also indicated if the child is doing well in all reality situations except one in which his poor functioning is due to environmental factors that cannot be altered.

There is one situation in which treatment ought to be brought to an end before it has run its planned course. If the child is completely uncooperative, it is not feasible to go on with therapy. If he is cooperative, but one or both of his parents are not, their attitudes will have to be explored before any decision is made on termination. It may be that they express only indifference or passive resentment, but are willing to shoulder the costs of treatment. In that event, further progress is possible if a good treatment relationship with the child has been formed. But there is little purpose in continuing if the parents are going through the motions of having their child treated solely in response to outside pressures, or if they are sabotaging the effort to create a constructive environment so effectively that their youngster has become very discouraged about his ability to modify his behavior.

SELECTED REFERENCES

Allen, F.: *Psychotherapy with Children.* New York, W. W. Norton, 1942.
Eysenck, H. J.: Learning theory and behavior therapy. *J. Ment. Sci.* 105:61-75, 1959.

Ford, D. H., and Urban, H. B.: *Systems of Psychotherapy*. New York, Wiley, 1963.

Freud, A.: *The Psychoanalytical Treatment of Children*. New York, International Universities Press, 1959.

Gondor, E. I.: *Art and Play Therapy*. New York, Doubleday, 1954.

Levy, D. M.: Release therapy. *Amer. J. Orthopsychiat.* 9:713-736, 1939.

Slavson, S. R.: *Analytic Group Psychotherapy*. New York, Columbia University Press, 1950.

Thomas, A., Chess, S., and Birch, H. G.: *Temperament and Behavior Disorders in Children*. New York, New York University Press, 1968.

Werry, J. S., and Wollersheim, J. P.: Behavior therapy with children: A broad overview. *J. Amer. Acad. Child Psychiat.* 6:346-370, 1967.

Wolpe, J.: *Psychotherapy by Reciprocal Inhibition*. Palo Alto, Stanford University Press, 1958.

17. Drug Therapy

THE USE OF DRUGS in the treatment of emotional disorders
has expanded tremendously during the past decade. In child
psychiatry, drugs have proved to be of considerable value and now
take precedence over all other forms of physiologic therapy. The
fully trained therapist must be familiar with a variety of medications, their application to the young patient, and their possible side
effects.

In some instances, drug treatment may be the only form of
psychiatric intervention required. More frequently, however, it
is employed in conjunction with other forms of treatment, usually
some kind of psychotherapy. If an organic illness is responsible for
a child's behavior problems, appropriate pharmacologic treatment
of the underlying disease will often modify the emotional difficulties. But if there is no identifiable organic disease and the behavioral
deviation is considered to be functional in origin, the choice of
a psychopharmacologic agent is based on the child's symptomatology.

Medication may be indicated in every category of behavioral
disorder. It may be useful for children with specific brain disorders,
systemic diseases in which disturbed behavior is one of the symptoms, and functional behavioral difficulties. Chief among the drugs
used in treating specific brain disorders are the anticonvulsants. A
classic example of drug therapy for a systemic disease process is
the administration of thyroid hormone, which usually alleviates
the behavior disturbance that may be one expression of thyroid
deficiency. In functional behavioral difficulties, drugs are mainly
used for their effect on symptoms.

In the treatment of certain symptoms, drugs may be particularly
useful. Thus, a child who displays hyperactivity, whether it is
physiologic, of neurologic origin, a symptom of cerebral dysfunction, or only fortuitously associated with mental retardation or
schizophrenia, should almost always be treated with an appropriate
psychopharmacologic agent (Stewart et al., 1966). The motoric

activity of a hyperactive child who is psychiatrically normal must be reduced and his attention span increased before he can experience a less stressful environment and start to benefit from instruction in school. If he has begun to show secondary behavioral symptoms, medication, perhaps combined with parent guidance or environmental manipulation, may be sufficient to induce a benign cycle in the child-environment interaction. Similarly, if a neurologic problem exists, medication may be necessary to lessen the annoying aspects of the child's disruptive hypermotility before the persons who make up his effective environment can begin to address themselves to relieving his difficulty; otherwise they have to focus exclusively on the destructive and disturbing consequences of the child's high energy level. This is also true when a hyperactive child has one of the more severe psychiatric disturbances. As long as the parents must be constantly alert to the disruption caused by the child, they cannot begin to train him. Once his hyperactivity is controlled, he may be amenable to the structuring of his behavior within the limits of his capacity to respond.

Another symptom that often requires psychopharmacologic intervention is anxiety, especially the child's subjective awareness of anxiety. It is sometimes necessary to decrease the anxiety associated wth a specific situation. For example, if a child refuses to go to school because of a phobic reaction, the use of psychopharmacologic agents may make it possible for him to return to class and to identify the anxiety-producing elements he finds within the school experience. Only then does it become possible to plan the appropriate therapeutic intervention dealing with the child's vulnerability to the offending element in the school situation. In some cases, anxiety leads to sleep disturbances, and the resultant fatigue interferes with the ability of the child, his family and the psychiatrist to work on the problem and to identify the precipitating cause of the anxiety. Here, too, the use of medications either to decrease anxiety specifically or to induce sleep may create circumstances more favorable to discussion of the emotional problem, since there will be less need to focus on the symptomatic representations of anxiety alone.

Depression is another symptom that sometimes demands a therapeutic attack with drugs. This is more likely to occur with adolescents than with younger children. Antidepressant medication may be required when a youngster is so preoccupied by his feelings of depression that he cannot identify the maladaptive elements of his daily life nor, for that matter, distinguish between events that evoke depressed feelings and events that are a consequence of depressed behavior.

When a behavioral problem is a symptom of an underlying disease, appropriate medication will, of course, be directed to the organic illness. As the disease responds to the medical regimen, one would anticipate an improvement in the child's behavioral manifestations. But symptoms that originally were reactive to the disease itself may sometimes develop an identity and continuity of their own, and psychotherapeutic intervention may be required for their alleviation. One must also keep in mind that medications used to treat an organic disease which has no behavioral manifestations may themselves cause behavioral changes. Thus, antihistamines may cause sleepiness and lethargy, and steroid therapy may result in the disorganization of behavior. If the child has a serious disease, and the medication is essential to its treatment, it may be necessary to continue drug therapy despite the behavioral aberrations it causes. If alternative medication exists, it is often advisable to change drugs. And if the organic disease is less disabling and destructive than the behavior changes that its treatment causes, it may be advisable to discontinue drug therapy.

Special Problems in Psychopharmacology

In administering medication to children, the physician must take into account the fact that many drugs act differently on children than on adults, and that some drugs may even have opposite effects. Children often require larger doses per unit of body weight than adults to obtain effective responses. In the following discussion, some average dosages will be specified. It should be emphasized, however, that dosages as well as the choice of medication may vary substantially from child to child.

Factors other than the choice of medication and dosage must also be considered. The reliability of the parents in carrying out directions may have a bearing on the results, as may the ability and willingness of the child to cooperate in taking the medicine. Thought should also be given to the form in which the medication is administered. Use of the parenteral route is actually the only way in which the physician can be sure that the child has received the drug in the prescribed dosage. Except in acute illness, however, the oral route is preferable, especially when medication must be given over a prolonged period of time. The physician must therefore face the fact that the cooperation of the child's parents and of the child himself is an important element in the effective use of drugs.

Even the best-intentioned parents may be forgetful about giving medicine or careless in measuring liquid preparations. Many parents are prone to seek additional opinions about the prescribed drugs, and become fearful about the dangers of the side reactions. All of these difficulties can be minimized by careful discussion with the parents when medication is begun.

The child's attitude is also crucial. He may be a generally negativistic youngster and thus be ready to sabotage any measure suggested to him by anyone. He may have a rebellious and hostile relationship with his mother, usually the person who administers the medicine. In this situation, taking the pill or liquid becomes a symbol of the struggle for domination between mother and child, and the youngster will find many ways to avoid swallowing his medicine. He may even, after a particularly violent altercation with his mother, take all the medicine in the bottle at one time as a retaliatory gesture. For this reason, it is often wisest to give prescriptions at weekly or biweekly intervals so that the amount of medication available in the home at any time is nonlethal.

The sabotaging child patient is adept at finding ways to avoid taking the prescribed medication. He may hide the pill between teeth and cheek and later on flush it down the toilet. Some children's institutions have had to revise their findings about the efficiency of drugs under study, because pills which had been recorded as successfully administered to the children were found under the rugs when they were taken up for the summer.

Such evasions and sabotage can be minimized by gaining the cooperation of the child. A more important reason for gaining his cooperation is that the best results are obtained when the patient comprehends what is being done and why it is being done. If the child has been distressed about his symptoms, the physician should explain to him in a straightforward way that the medicine will lessen these symptoms. The explanation must, of course, be given in terms suitable for the child's age and intellectual level. Even a young child can be made to understand that the medicine will help him. An older child's interest can be secured by giving him some responsibility for watching the clock and keeping track of the correct timing of his medication. A hyperactive child, for example, can be motivated to cooperate in taking his medicine if he understands that it will help him sit still long enough at school to learn something and free him from the teacher's constant scolding.

The form in which medication can best be administered also needs careful consideration. For young children who cannot swallow pills or capsules, one may use liquid preparations or solid preparations that have been crushed and sugared. The staggered release capsule is a useful form if a sustained blood level of the medication is desirable. Another advantage of such capsules is that one morning dose is all that is required for a period of twelve hours, and the child does not have to carry a pill to school to be swallowed—or more likely not swallowed—during his lunch hour.

The final choice of the specific medication must be made on an empiric basis. Some children respond to the first drug administered. With other children, the physician must try one drug after another before obtaining the optimum therapeutic response with minimal side effects.

Psychopharmacologic Agents for Children

Anticonvulsants

Even though an epileptic child who is subject to frequent convulsions may also manifest hyperactivity, irritability, negativism and an inability to concentrate, the choice of his medication is generally determined by the underlying organic disease. The restlessness or confusional state that is secondary to the convulsive disorder is controlled by adequate anticonvulsant medication.

Of the barbiturates, *phenobarbital* is most commonly used for children with convulsive disorders. The dosage of phenobarbital will be determined by the difficulty of controlling the convulsions, but 15 to 30 mg. three times a day is considered average.

Diphenylhydantoin (Dilantin) may also be used for behavior disorders in which an epileptic equivalence is suspected. It is frequently useful in ameliorating hyperirritability and hyperactivity of both functional and organic (convulsive) origin. However, because of secondary manifestations, such as hypertrophy of the gums and ataxia, it should not be the medication of choice where there is no suspicion of convulsive disorder. For children under six years of age, the average dosage is .03 to .3 Gm. t.i.d. For children over six, the average dose is .1 Gm. t.i.d.

Sedatives

Barbiturates (especially *phenobarbital*) are sometimes used to help with sleep problems. However, they may have the paradoxic effect of exciting rather than quieting the child, in which case they should be discontinued.

Chloral hydrate is useful for children whose inability to fall asleep is serious enough to merit pharmacologic intervention. The child should be given approximately 50 to 75 mg. at bedtime. Antihistamines may also be used to sedate children.

Drugs with Tranquilizing Effects

Antihistamines have been used beneficially to reduce activity level, subjective feelings of anxiety and, at times, compulsive behaviors. *Diphenhydramine HCL* (Benadryl) is particularly useful with children and is usually given in pill or liquid form in doses of 10 to 20 mg. t.i.d. *Promethazine HCL* (Phenergan) is another frequently used antihistamine.

Phenothiazines have been successfully used in children with a variety of behavior disorders as well as for controlling muscular tics. As part of a total therapeutic plan, *chlorpromazine* (Thorazine) may be used to reduce anxiety in children who have phobic reactions to school attendance or in youngsters who have a high anxiety level which erupts into fearfulness at many points during the daily activities. In some cases, too, it may be useful in decreasing a youngster's activity level. Thorazine *is* available in syrup or tablet form. Pediatric dosages range from 5 to 75 or 100 mg. daily, depending upon the age and size of the child.

Trifluoperazine (Stelazine) is also useful with hyperactive schizophrenic or neurotic children. It is particularly recommended for psychotic children, and has been reported to increase their ability to respond to interpersonal advances and demands for attentiveness to programmed activities. The usual dose is 1 mg. once or twice a day, but schizophrenic children can tolerate up to 15 mg. daily.

The phenothiazines may induce extrapyramidal symptoms, including the muscular rigidity and tremor of Parkinson's syndrome, as well as the upward rolling of the eyes and the oculogyric crises usually associated with a chronic postencephalitic neurologic disorder.

To relieve the extrapyramidal symptoms, none of which are in themselves dangerous, it is recommended that either the medication be stopped or that it be continued in conjunction with one of the antiparkinsonism drugs, such as *trihexyphenidyl HCL* (Artane) 5 mg. b.i.d. or *benztropine methansulfonate* (Cogentin) 1 mg. b.i.d.

Prochlorperazine (Compazine) is widely used interchangeably with *chlorpromazine*. However, of all the phenothiazines this drug is particularly capable of producing extrapyramidal symptoms in children, and its use should therefore be avoided. Prochlorperazine reportedly has caused such symptoms as tongue thrust and stiffening of the jaw muscles. Intravenous Benadryl is a specific antidote to the prochlorperazine reaction.

Agranulocytosis, which has been reported as a rare complication in adults taking phenothiazines, has not as yet been reported in children. Nevertheless, a blood count should be taken before the drug is administered as well as periodically thereafter so that a falling white count can be immediately identified. The appearance of frequent upper respiratory infections or delay in the healing of minor skin infections should also be a signal for investigating the possibility of leucocytopenia. In addition, though liver damage has not been reported in children, youngsters receiving phenothiazines should be routinely observed for signs of early jaundice. And, since sensitivity to sunlight has been found as another side reaction, these drugs should be used with considerable care during the summer so as to avoid the possibility of heat exhaustion and shock.

Amphetamines, though minor stimulants, have often been reported to have a paradoxic effect when administered to prepubertal,
hyperactive children. They decrease the youngster's activity level
and distractibility while they increase his attention span. The
dextroamphetamine form of the drug is most commonly employed.
Dosages vary from 5 mg. t.i.d. in a younger child to 10 mg. q.i.d. in
a ten or eleven year old. If there are signs of beginning puberty, the
use of amphetamines should be discontinued, as one would tend to
get the more familiar stimulating effects seen in adults. Side
reactions include dryness of the mouth, temporary loss of appetite
and interference with sleep. If the child's sleeplessness becomes a
problem, it may be necessary to stop the medication. However, if
the last dose of the drug is given at 4 P.M. or earlier, it is not
likely to keep the child awake.

Methylphenidate (Ritalin) is considered by some investigators to
be the drug of choice for hyperactive children. This agent has
relatively few side effects. The dosage is 5 to 10 mg. t.i.d.

Meprobamate (Equanil, Miltown) is of value in lessening apprehension and anxiety level. It can also be used to help induce sleep
in children whose insomnia is caused by fears. The average pediatric dosage is approximately 100 mg., one to three times a day,
and amounts up to 400 mg. are not considered unduly large.

Imipramine (Tofrānil) is of use in some cases for lowering anxiety
level and decreasing activity level. It has been particularly effective
in reducing the frequency of nocturnal enuresis.

Chlordiazepoxide (Librium) and *diazepam* (Valium) may also be
used as tranquilizers for children. And, since they have been reported to be muscle relaxants, they may have special use in controlling tics. Initial dosages for children would be 5 mg. *chlordiazepoxide* and 2 mg. *diazepam.*

Haloperidol (Haldol) has been reported to be effective in controlling childhood tics, and especially in the Maladie de Gilles de
la Tourette, in which there are multiple muscular tics, a bark-like
cough, and explosive coprolalia. While some cases of this disease
have responded to phenothiazine or chlordiazepoxide, the effects of
haloperidol have been most striking. However, at the present time,
this drug has been approved for use only in children over twelve
years of age.

Since depressions are difficult to identify in children, antidepressant drugs are not usually given. With adolescents one would use the same drugs as in adults, including the amphetamines and *amitriptyline HCL* (Elavil). However, in prescribing amphetamines for adolescents one must take into account the possibility of drug abuse and addiction.

Other Physiologic Therapies

Shock therapy, although rarely used in the treatment of children, should be noted as one form of physiologic treatment. Schizophrenic children with disorganized and hyperkinetic behavior patterns have been reported by some investigators as becoming more organized for a period of time in response to a course of electroshock treatment. This therapy may be carried out as an office procedure as well as in the hospital. Approximately twenty shocks are given, spaced from one to several days apart. Child psychiatrists in general are reluctant, in the present state of knowledge in this area, to utilize shock therapy in the treatment of children.

Finally, one should note that insulin shock therapy and lobotomy have been tried in the past but, since neither proved of particular use, these treatment measures are not used at all with children today and are only of historical interest.

SELECTED REFERENCES

Bender, L., and Nichtern, S.: Chemotherapy in child psychiatry. *New York State J. Med.* 56:2791-2795, 1956.

Bradley, C.: Benzedrine and dexedrine in the treatment of children's behavior disorders. *Pediatrics* 5:24-37, 1950.

Eisenberg, L. et al.: A psychopharmacologic experiment in a training school for delinquent boys. *Amer. J. Orthopsychiat.* 33:431-447, 1963.

Fish, B.: Drug use in psychiatric disorders of children. *Amer. J. Psychiat.* 124:31-36, 1968.

Laufer, M. W.: Amphetamines in organic brain disease. *Psychosom. Med.* 19:38-49, 1957.

Poussaint, A. F., and Ditman, K. S.: A controlled study of Imipramine (Tofranil) in the treatment of childhood enuresis. *J. Pediat.* 67:283-290, 1965.

Shaw, C. R. et al.: Tranquilizer drugs in the treatment of emotionally disturbed children. *J. Amer. Acad. Child Psychiat.* 2:725, 1963.

Stewart, M. A. et al.: The hyperactive child syndrome. *Amer. J. Orthopsychiat.* 36:861-867, 1966.

18. Inpatient and Outpatient Treatment

SOME CHILDREN who require psychiatric treatment are best cared for as inpatients in a special institution, others as outpatients in a clinic or in private practice. The decision depends on the nature and severity of a child's illness and the specific circumstances of his environment.

Most emotionally disturbed children who receive treatment live in their own homes, foster homes or child-care centers. In general, it is better for the child to remain in his normal environment than to live in a psychiatric hospital or other institution while undergoing therapy. As an outpatient, the child is spared the trauma of separation from his family, or at least from accustomed surroundings. It becomes possible to study and handle difficulties in the child's environment, particularly child-parent interactions, during treatment. It is also easier to achieve the goal of a good adjustment in the home, school, and community.

Outpatient Treatment

Outpatient psychiatric treatment for children is given in clinics of various types, most often entitled "child guidance clinics," and in private practice. The clinics function either in hospital settings as one of a number of outpatient services, or as units organized and supported by state or municipal mental hygiene departments, churches and social agencies. As opposed to adult psychiatry, in which there are very few differences between the procedures followed by clinics and by private practitioners, child guidance clinics have developed a special organizational structure for intake and diagnosis of patients.

In most clinics, the procedural pattern involves an interdisciplinary team, basically comprising a psychiatrist, a psychologist and a social worker. Some clinics also include pediatricians, nurses, educators, speech therapists and other specialists as members of the team. The precise service performed by each member and the specific disciplines represented vary from clinic to clinic, according to the center's treatment philosophy, its affiliation, the extent to which it can use other community resources and the special needs of its patients.

When a child is referred to a typical psychiatric clinic, he goes through a complicated "intake" process. Usually, he is first placed on a waiting list for a turn to be evaluated. When an opening occurs, sometimes as much as a year later, the conventional procedure is for a social worker to take the admission history; a psychologist then administers a battery of tests, and a psychiatrist conducts a clinical examination.

The histories taken by the social worker in different institutions vary widely in content and focus, depending on the clinic's theoretic framework and its concept of what elements are most important for diagnostic consideration. Thus, the social worker may dwell on such aspects of the situation as the parents' attitudes, the sequence of events in the child's life, facts about the parents' lives, and the child's behavioral difficulties. While some clinics do psychologic testing routinely in all cases, others use these procedures selectively. Routine testing is generally done before the initial interview with the child, though it may also be done afterward. The psychiatrist, too, may vary his procedure by arranging for a discussion with the parents, as well as the child, to supplement the social worker's interview. In addition, pediatric examinations and other consultations may be scheduled when necessary.

When all of these data have been obtained, a diagnostic formulation will be made by the interdisciplinary team—psychiatrist, psychologist and social worker—in joint discussion. In some clinics, other professional personnel who have examined the child participate in the discussion, while in other clinics they submit their findings to the basic team. The final diagnosis is a medical one, made by the psychiatrist, who also makes the decision to accept the child for therapy. If it is concluded that the clinic can give service appropriate to the child's needs, the team makes detailed plans for his treatment, although usually the child must again be placed on a waiting list. Usually, the parents are referred to the social worker for continuing case work and the child is treated by a psychiatrist or by a nonmedical psychotherapist working under the psychiatrist's supervision. If the particular case seems to warrant it, the parents may receive psychiatric treatment or the child may be seen by the social worker under case work procedure. Moreover, since a significant proportion of the children seen in guidance clinics function academically below the level of their intellectual capacity, many clinics provide remedial-education services. This work is done by psychologists or special instructors.

As treatment proceeds, staff personnel who deal with various aspects of the child's problems correlate their results through regularly scheduled conferences. The therapist receives reports on the child's behavior, on alterations in his environment, and on the attitudes toward the child of the significant persons in his life. The social worker is informed of the problems that emerge in treatment, and utilizes this information in his work with the parents. The remedial-education worker gives pertinent data about the youngster's difficulties and successes, and receives information that helps him gear his approach to the child's needs and capacities.

This standard procedure has a number of drawbacks. First of all, the long waiting lists both for treatment and evaluation prevent one from giving a child immediate attention at the time of referral. Secondly, since not every child requires the extensive and involved work-up routinely advised, time and manpower are wasted. Third, by almost universally recommending psychotherapy, clinics often get bogged down in unnecessarily lengthy courses of treatment that are not always best for a particular child. Finally, there are wide variations in the degree to which the disciplines function cooperatively. Too often the traditional hierarchy of the surgical or medical team is uncritically taken over, with the psychiatrist in command and members of all other disciplines considered ancillary personnel. A strict hierarchic set-up tends to minimize the contribution of the social worker and psychologist, and may impede full use of the data revealed by their work.

To overcome the drawbacks of the standard approach, a few clinics have made some significant innovations. These clinics are set up to see a child immediately when a consultation is requested, to obtain a quick diagnostic judgment, to arrange promptly for further work-ups, and to plan an individualized treatment program. Among the clinics taking this approach are those at the Yale

Child Study Center in New Haven and at Bellevue Hospital in New York.

The psychiatric department at Bellevue, as part of a growing awareness of the need for community mental health care, has organized a psychiatric unit in the pediatric outpatient department (Chess and Lyman, 1969). The unit deals with referrals from the pediatric or other specialty clinic, the social service department, or various community schools or agencies. Within minutes after referral, the child and his parents are seen by either a psychiatrist, psychologist, or psychiatric social worker on the special clinic team. There is no standard intake procedure. Instead, an immediate screening process has been designed for determining quickly if a psychiatric problem exists. If it does, recommendations are made at once for emergency measures or further work-ups. The goal of the work-up is to establish a diagnosis and define a plan of management. Children do not automatically get the same work-up; the schedule of procedures is individually determined. Treatment techniques are also varied, again depending on the specific nature of the case. The methods used include parent guidance, other environmental manipulation, recreational play group activity, remedial education, and individual or group psychotherapy for child or parent.

Clearly, whether a clinic takes this new approach or a more traditional one will be determined in part by its theoretic goals. Also important, although not so clearly recognized, are such factors as the clinic's geographic locale, the cultural and racial backgrounds of the children, and the socioeconomic groups to which they belong. These factors must be taken into account in diagnostic and treatment procedures.

An example of a clinic in a crowded urban area is the Northside Center for Child Development in New York. The Center, located in Harlem, serves families whose financial status ranges from dependence on home relief to middle class, and whose racial and cultural backgrounds differ widely. The problems this clinic encounters and the techniques it uses obviously differ from those of a child guidance clinic which serves a more homogeneous group. To meet the challenge of understanding the children and their parents despite linguistic and cultural differences, the staff is interracial, intercultural and multilingual, with skills and approaches that might not be required in another setting. For example, it pioneered in providing special remedial education as a therapeutic instrument for children whose emotional problems were such that they could not make use of ordinary remedial work. It was found that this procedure was a way of giving a child a sense of personal dignity that then allowed him to deal more effectively with the problems of formal education and learning.

Clinic practice contrasts with private practice, where the psychiatrist acts alone rather than as a member of an interdisciplinary team. Usually he deals with the parents in obtaining the initial history and in providing whatever therapy and support are indicated. In addition, he himself makes contact with school personnel and other significant persons for information and assistance in working out plans for the child's treatment. Some private practitioners, however, do have close working relationships with one or more psychologists or a private social worker, and these professional workers expedite his work for him. Certainly, the psychiatrist in private practice has an advantage in that he obtains all the information he needs himself, without losing time waiting for others to do their assignments. Yet the very nature of his solo practice may keep him from making optimum use of community facilities, for both diagnosis and treatment, and, in some specific cases, this may be to the disadvantage of the child patient.

Inpatient Treatment

Certain kinds and degrees of emotional disturbance indicate the need for inpatient care. Among those requiring it are children who respond to anxiety by suicidal attempts, as well as those who become extremely aggressive or resort to dangerous impulsive acts. For the child whose home environment reinforces the basic problem, milieu therapy in a residential setting may be indicated.

Inpatient psychiatric treatment, however, should be recommended only when it is the treatment of choice. It should not be used in lieu of adequate foster home care or simply because other forms of treatment have failed. One must carefully analyze the reasons for such failure and undertake corrective measures, instead of automatically sending a child off to an institution. If parental handling has been so capricious, neglectful or destructive that the child cannot profit by outpatient treatment, this situation should be met by placing the child in a foster home or normal child-care institution, not by prescribing inpatient treatment. It must be remembered that institutional psychiatric care is a specialized and relatively temporary service, a specific experience that aims to return the child to the environment provided for him in his own home, through foster care, or in some other way.

Sometimes, inpatient treatment is clearly indicated as the treatment of choice, but cannot be provided because the child's parents are unwilling to agree to institutional care. In such cases, a compromise plan is obviously better than none at all. Under such an arrangement, a clinic would accept the child for treatment having a modified goal—that is, a goal that would fall short of what might be expected for a full program of inpatient treatment. It is quite possible that after some progress has been made, the parents may alter their attitude and consent to inpatient treatment. It is also possible that the results will be better than had been anticipated, since the criteria for deciding upon inpatient or outpatient treatment are by no means always clear-cut and well-defined.

Under certain circumstances, residential treatment may be the treatment of choice in any diagnostic category. The child with a reactive or a moderate neurotic behavior disorder who is being subjected to neglectful or destructive handling at home may make a speedier recovery in an institution that provides a favorable environment. Children with more severe difficulties may need the planned regime and special approaches provided in an institutional setting while undergoing treatment.

In the very severe diagnostic categories, such as sociopathic personality, childhood schizophrenia, retardation and extreme deviant behavior, institutional treatment may be necessary. Many schizophrenic children can best be started on the road to adequate social development in a residential setting. This is not true, however, in all cases of childhood schizophrenia, and first consideration should be given to outpatient treatment.

The behavior of the extremely deviant child may be so inimical to the legitimate needs of his siblings and parents, who are after all "people" as well as parents, that to keep the child at home imposes needless stress on the family with no gain for the patient. The wisest course may be institutional treatment aiming at remission of the difficulty. In some cases, an indefinite period of custodial care may be indicated.

Residential treatment may be the best way of handling the delinquent child who is caught in a vicious cycle in which the only peer group that accepts him is a delinquent group. The experience of institutional living plus psychiatric treatment may well be the only way to bring about a change in this child's behavioral pattern. Another child may be caught up in a negative interaction that cannot be handled at home. His demoralization about schoolwork, for example, is leading to hooky-playing and delinquency. In a residential setting, his educational problem can be dealt with more objectively than if he were home and his parents were constantly having to police him.

Similarly, in the development of a child there may arise a time of impending disaster, and this, even more than the basic diagnosis, requires that he be institutionalized. In such cases, it may prove impossible to control the home environment effectively—for example, when a parent is undergoing an acute psychiatric crisis which is creating disorganization in the home and acting out on the child's part. Sometimes, a child will be best treated residentially at one age and not at another, even though his basic pathology remains the same. Thus, a mentally retarded child may be achieving up to his intellectual capacity at home, but because of his deficiency he is kept from participating in any semblance of a social life. Temporary residential treatment in his school years may give him the necessary opportunity for peer relationships, and the experience of social life will make it possible for him to return home in young adulthood and function in a healthy, social manner.

In some cases, it is parental intransigence that necessitates inpatient treatment of a child. For instance, if a mother refuses to bring her child for treatment of a perceptual disorder or some other defect, he may eventually develop secondary emotional problems. Although these, too, could be treated in an outpatient clinic, the mother's continued refusal to bring the child may become the deciding factor in recommending inpatient care. In other instances, a child who has been physically abused by his parents must be removed from them. If the child has developed a behavior disorder in response to this injurious handling, it may be necessary to place him in a special institution. If his emotional pathology is minimal, foster home care or cottage living may be appropriate treatment. The new environment must be chosen on the basis of what has happened to the child's behavior and what circumstances would be most ameliorative. In all these examples, inpatient care is indicated because the expectation is that psychiatric treatment will be more effective under the living conditions provided by the institution than under the living conditions of outpatient care.

In addition, there are those children for whom institutional care of a custodial nature is mandatory. In these cases, the child's psychiatric state may be such that he cannot be managed in his home environment. The youngster may be so retarded or so unpredictable that it is impossible to plan a constructive program for him, or he may be dangerous to himself and others. While such children often cannot be helped by therapeutic inpatient care, they nevertheless require custodial attention.

Inpatient Facilities

The earliest inpatient facilities tended to be for children who were mentally retarded, or at least those who were judged to be retarded. Most of these institutions began as custodial centers, places to "dump" incorrigibles. During the 20th century, however, the possibility of returning at least some of these children to society began to be acknowledged. Institutions were then established not merely to isolate but to treat children. At the present time, emphasis is on the expansion of both foster care programs (for the reasons discussed earlier in this chapter) and institutional facilities. Unfortunately, the demand for inpatient treatment has increased faster than the number of available centers. As a result, there is now an enormous backlog of children awaiting placement, sometimes for as long as two or three years. In hardship situations, these children are placed in foster homes until they can be institutionalized. But even foster home facilities cannot absorb the waiting children as well as those for whom such placement is the treatment of choice.

There is, in addition, a group of children living as "boarders" in hospitals. Many of these have remained because parents failed to take them home after birth or after a subsequent hospitalization. In many such cases, the children have birth defects and are retarded. Their parents may be drug addicts or sociopaths, and the lengthy stay in a hospital is due to the absence of a responsible person who can authorize placement in a foster home or institution. The relevance for psychiatry is that these youngsters spend months or years in the very type of impersonal institutional care likely to create personality disorder.

Inpatient psychiatric treatment for children is provided in many types of centers. These may be units of state hospitals, general or psychiatric hospitals; or they may be privately sponsored, autonomous institutions. They are supported by public funds—municipal, state or federal—or by private funds. Sometimes they derive their support from a combination of sources. All the centers are medical facilities in which psychiatrists carry medical responsibility for the diagnosis and treatment of the child. Emphasis is on treatment through psychotherapy, somatic therapies and the living setting—sometimes called milieu therapy—with the goal of returning the child to the community.

Other types of institutions place their emphasis on continuing care for disturbed children who cannot be reared in their own homes or in foster homes. The extremely deviant child may have to be placed in such an institution for custodial care. The severely retarded child may best be cared for in a center for retarded children. Children with serious physical handicaps, such as cerebral palsy or orthopedic difficulties of extreme severity, may require indefinite institutional care.

Institutions for inpatient treatment and care of children vary widely in the size of their patient population, their physical set-up, their policies regarding admission of children in various diagnostic categories, and in many other ways. A cottage-type set-up may be the entire format or a part of it, and even institutions with several hundred youngsters often consider it best to divide them into small groups of from ten to twenty. Sometimes these groups are under the care of a cottage mother or of a couple who presumably act as surrogate parents. Grouping may be by chronologic age, intellectual age, type of difficulty, or according to some other scheme. It should be noted, however, that there still are many large institutions that have only a ward plan.

In general, children's facilities in state hospitals have the largest number of patients, while autonomous private centers have the smallest. The ratio of personnel to patients also varies, with low ratios in state hospitals and other public institutions and high ratios in private centers. There are, of course, exceptions to this general statement. Some centers, especially the larger ones, have intramural schools, with teachers assigned by the community public school system or employed by the parent organization. A few of the smaller centers use community school facilities. Some centers have a combined educational set-up in which community schooling is supplemented by special educational work within the institution, according to the children's needs.

The problem of selecting an institution is complicated when the child has multiple disabilities. In these cases, one frequently must decide which is the outstanding or target defect. For example, if a mentally retarded child also has a convulsive disorder, he may be accepted at an institution for retardates. However, if the convulsive disorder is the major management problem, he may have to be placed in a specialized inpatient facility that is oriented more toward handling this difficulty. Similarly, if a child has both an emotional and a physical problem, the latter may limit either the number of places that will accept him or the number of places that are best suited to meet his specific needs. In every case, subsidiary and major problems must be distinguished and given appropriate weight in selecting an institution. An extensive listing of residential schools, clinics and hospitals is provided in the publication, *Directory for Exceptional Children* (Sargent, 1965). This helpful handbook includes a capsule summary of the number and kind of children accepted, the remedial and vocational facilities available, the living arrangements and fees.

In residential treatment centers that accept children with varying psychiatric disorders, management approaches must be flexible enough to be pertinent to each youngster. An outstanding example of such an institution is Hawthorne Center in Northville, Michigan (Shaw, 1966). This center provides both day and boarding facilities, cottage as well as ward living. Hawthorne has its own school. While the children are grouped according to their approximate academic level, there are also provisions for individual plans of study and tutoring. In addition to individual sessions with a psychiatrist, each child receives therapeutic support and education from a team of specialists including language therapists, occupational therapists, social workers, psychiatric nurses and specially trained teachers.

Effects of Inpatient Treatment

It is difficult to predict what the effect of residential treatment will be in any given case. The hope that it will foster some degree of improvement in the child's condition must be balanced against the fact that in some cases separation from the family may be overridingly disadvantageous. Sending a child to a treatment and education center does not change the diagnosis or remake the child. Nevertheless, it is possible to get the optimum behavior of which he is capable by the pertinent organization of the available services. The retarded child will stay retarded, but he can be educated to assume some degree of responsibility for himself. The emotionally disturbed child may continue to have personality problems, but it does pay to attempt to socialize him and develop his capacity for responsiveness. These children need not automatically be written off and hidden away.

Obviously, purely custodial care will not produce these changes and may, in fact, have certain deleterious effects. The most severe of these is "hospitalism" (Spitz, 1945), a term referring to the psychologic deprivation of infants in hospitals. In the past, institutional life was indeed emotionally and perceptually sterile, but many new approaches have been taken to enrich residential facilities. Foremost among these is cottage living, which attempts to give inpatients an approximation of home life. Most institutions which do not consider themselves to have a strictly custodial function try to widen the child's opportunities for social and educational experiences. Many residential centers schedule visits by the child to his family on weekends or during vacations, so that he maintains some contact with his normal environment. Although it cannot be denied that institutionalized children do not always fare as well as children in outpatient treatment in a number of ways (institutionalized retardates, for example, have consistently poorer language functioning than do those living at home), we have progressed from the bedlams of the past and have at least acknowledged the need for improvement.

SELECTED REFERENCES

Alt, H.: *Residential Treatment for the Disturbed Child.* New York, International Universities Press, 1960.

American Psychiatric Association: *Psychiatric Inpatient Treatment of Children (1956 Conference).* Washington, American Psychiatric Association, 1957.

Chess, S., and Lyman, M.: A psychiatric unit in a general hospital pediatric clinic. *Amer. J. Orthopsychiat.* 39:77-85, 1969.

Chess, S., and Rubin, E.: Treatment of schizophrenic children in a child guidance clinic. *Nervous Child,* 10:167-178, 1952.

Hylton, L. F.: *The Residential Treatment Center.* New York, Child Welfare League of America, 1964.

Shaw, C. R.: *The Psychiatric Disorders of Childhood.* New York, Appleton-Century-Crofts, 1966.

Sargent, P.: *The Directory for Exceptional Children.* Boston, Porter Sargent, 1965.

Spitz, R. A.: Hospitalism: An inquiry into the genesis of psychiatric conditions in early childhood. *Psychoanalytic Study of the Child,* Vol. 1. New York, International Universities Press, 1945.

Index

258

INDEX